THE FIBROMYALGIA HANDBOOK

THE
FIBROMYALGIA
HANDBOOK

A 7-Step Program to Halt and Even Reverse Fibromyalgia

HARRIS H. McILWAIN, M.D.
DEBRA FULGHUM BRUCE, M.S.

Third Edition

AN OWL BOOK
HENRY HOLT AND COMPANY
NEW YORK

Henry Holt and Company, LLC
Publishers since 1866
115 West 18th Street
New York, New York 10011

Henry Holt® is a registered trademark of
Henry Holt and Company, LLC.

Library of Congress Cataloging-in-Publication Data

McIlwain, Harris H.
    The fibromyalgia handbook : a 7-step program to halt
    and even reverse fibromyalgia / Harris H. McIlwain
    and Debra Fulghum Bruce.—3rd ed.
        p.   cm.
    "An Owl book."
    Includes index.
    ISBN 0-8050-7241-1 (pbk.)
    1. Fibromyalgia—Handbooks, manuals, etc.
    I. Bruce, Debra Fulghum, date. II. Title.

RC927.3 .M36 2003
616.7'4—dc21   2002027492

Henry Holt books are available for special promotions
and premiums. For details contact: Director, Special Markets.

First Edition 1996
Second Edition 1999
Third Edition 2003

Designed by Ann Gold
Illustrations on pages 124, 125, 127, and 128 are by James Russell, M.S.

Printed in the United States of America

10   9   8   7   6   5   4   3   2   1

CONTENTS

THE FIBROMYALGIA HANDBOOK

INTRODUCTION: YOU HAVEN'T GOT TIME FOR THE PAIN

As a board certified rheumatologist, I've treated thousands of patients over the past twenty-five years. I'm part of Tampa Medical Group; we have three large pain clinics on Florida's pristine Gulf Coast and see hundreds of patients each week.

Because I diagnose and treat men and women with fibro-myalgia daily, I am passionate about finding new treatments for this epidemic problem. Some of these therapies include break-through medications that help to end pain and give you back your active life. Others are as simple as the over-the-counter dietary supplement SAM-e, a deep-muscle massage, or certain yoga postures.

If you have been diagnosed with fibromyalgia, fibrositis, or myofascial pain syndrome, no one needs to tell you of the almost daily muscle pain you live with, along with constant fatigue, sleeplessness, and low-grade depression. I've seen fibromyalgia take its toll on once healthy individuals, especially women ages twenty to sixty. Not only does it strike during the young and middle adult years—the busiest and most stressful time of one's life, but patients tell of the symptoms making them feel as if they are a hundred years old. The good news is that *it does not have to be this way!* You can live actively with fibromyalgia, *if* you learn how to manage its symptoms.

Years ago, it became apparent to doctors that patients who told of having muscle aches, fatigue, depression, headaches, and sleeplessness were harboring a distinct disease or syndrome (a collection of symptoms that make a disease). Yet the results from lab tests and X rays were always normal. Two decades ago, physicians sent these patients home with few answers, as we could only treat the symptoms.

Today we know differently. In the past five years there has been a plethora of research done on this mysterious syndrome we call "fibromyalgia" or FMS. Now millions of people can understand that the disease is real; the symptoms are *not* imagined *nor* did they cause them; and treatment does work, if followed faithfully.

A View of Fibromyalgia

In this book, you will become knowledgeable about fibromyalgia and learn how to lessen the severity of the symptoms. Questions will be addressed, such as:

- Does being overweight make one more likely to get fibromyalgia?
- Why is this considered a "female" disease?
- Does estrogen have anything to do with it?
- Is there a cure for this or will it continue to cause pain for my entire life?
- Should I push myself on days when the pain and fatigue seem unbearable?
- How do I know which medications will help me?
- How can I know for sure that this is fibromyalgia?
- Will the disease run its course?
- Did I cause the disease from too much stress or poor nutrition?
- Did an injury cause it?
- Does exercise hurt or help the painful symptoms?
- Is it inherited?

While there are no cures for fibromyalgia, you can learn to control your specific symptoms as you manage the disease with the 7-Step Treatment Program. This plan has proved to be successful with thousands of my patients as they identify the symptoms of the disease, carefully seek a diagnosis, and learn to manage the disease in a reasonable way.

Let's look at some patients who have taken the steps needed to control their fibromyalgia and are winning with this disease.

Chronic Fatigue and Muscle Pain

Linda was one patient who benefited greatly from the combination 7-Step Treatment Program outlined in this book. After her youngest child entered elementary school, this thirty-nine-year-old woman enrolled at the local university to work on her master's degree. Halfway through the quarter, Linda noticed a dramatic change in her health. "I've always needed eight hours of sleep," she said upon evaluation. "But for the past month, I have been sleeping eleven or twelve hours and still feel tired when I awaken."

This once active woman told of feeling so chronically fatigued that even walking to class from a nearby parking lot left her feeling weak. She said that even a cool breeze on her skin felt like burning fire and the only relief she could get from this pain was lying down in bed. "Imagine feeling like you had worked out for hours, yet all you did was make your breakfast and take a shower."

After seeing three physicians, including a sleep disorders specialist who ruled out any nighttime respiratory problems, Linda came to our clinic. In the meantime, Linda continued to take courses while maintaining a family. But the added stress of going to school and studying took its toll, for she felt overwrought, as if her body was failing her.

Upon diagnosis, Linda began the 7-Step Treatment Program, including a specific focus on dietary changes (see chapter 9), stress reduction, and gentle stretching exercises several times a day. As predicted, her symptoms responded positively. Within three weeks, Linda felt relief from the constant, nagging pain and was able to increase her normal activity.

Hot, Searing Leg Pain

Jean, a high school principal, told of being unable to walk one morning about five years ago. "I'll never forget that day for as long as I live. I had set my alarm early that morning because the accreditation team was coming to the school for our annual review.

"When I put my feet on the floor, my legs simply gave way. My left ankle had a hot, searing, and burning pain that went throughout the heel, arch, and toes. When I sat on my right hip, my thigh and leg hurt so badly, it was unbearable. There was a pinching feeling in my hip and I could hardly walk. All I could think of was that my career was over."

After a CT (computerized tomography) scan and MRI (magnetic resonance imaging)—two commonly used imaging techniques to see inside the body—showed no medical reason for her pain, Jean came to our clinic for an evaluation. She had been told by two doctors that her pain was a mental health problem, yet as an educator, she knew there was more to it. In fact, her symptoms of pain and fatigue were so relentless that it took several months to get this under control.

As Linda and thousands have experienced, once Jean received the diagnosis of fibromyalgia and began the treatment program, she was able to increase activity and live a normal life again.

Achiness, Fatigue, and Depression

When Elizabeth, a forty-five-year-old attorney, got over a recent bout with the flu, she thought that the achiness that lingered was from being run down. "I had this unending pain that made me so depressed. I even thought that death would be a welcome relief, because I hurt all over. The pain became so intense that I couldn't have sex with my husband without tears, yet he did not seem to understand. I couldn't even do light household chores without wanting to scream out in agony."

It took three months of doctors' appointments until Elizabeth's symptoms were finally given a name—fibromyalgia. "How could doctors look me straight in the eye and say that the pain and fatigue were in my head? One doctor said that a cruise would make me feel less stressed. A cruise? I didn't need a cruise, I needed a diagnosis, and, more important, I needed a form of treatment."

For Elizabeth, living with fibromyalgia has been an eye-opening experience. "It is hard to realize that healthy people can get this disease, but they can. I now understand that education is the key in controlling the symptoms."

Most important, the quality of life for Linda, Jean, and Elizabeth has greatly improved since starting the treatment plan. All three tell of now sleeping soundly, having more energy, and feeling less pressure since they took control of the debilitating symptoms.

The reactions of other men and women who successfully halted or even reversed fibromyalgia on the 7-Step Treatment Program are just as encouraging:

- Paul, age forty-one, with deep muscle pain in his thighs, lower back, and shoulders, said, "I learned to cut back on unnecessary commitments and now use that time to take care of myself. It was difficult at first because I felt so selfish, spending my evenings exercising and enjoying my CD collection with friends. The exercise and relaxation help me to calm down and sleep well, so I wake up feeling refreshed and with less muscle pain. I've also added more fresh fruits and vegetables to my diet, and go to the farmers' market in our town each Saturday to stock up on the best produce. I'm taking one of the new COX-2 medications, which helps to ease muscle aches. To be honest, I never thought I'd feel good again, and I now do almost anything I want."

- Mira, age twenty-three, with chronic neck pain, migraines, and TMJ (temporomandibular joint) syndrome, said, "I use the warm Jacuzzi at my condo before I go to work and during the evening hours. Not only does the heat ease the muscle pain, but also I feel so relaxed that my sleep quality has greatly improved. I wake up smiling now, ready to take on the day. I started a yoga class at work and do the postures daily to stretch my sore muscles. Over-the-counter Advil seems to help, so now I exercise without fear of more pain."

- Luci, age thirty-seven, with deep muscle pain in her thighs and lower back, said, "I feel ten years younger after starting this program and finally feel in control of my life—and my pain. Each of the seven steps is designed to help you control one area of your life—from your physical activity to your diet to your sleep to your stress levels. I've learned to demand less of myself and others, and now I enjoy the little things in life more."

- Jim, age fifty-two, with deep muscle pain in his shoulders and neck and osteoarthritis in his hip, said, "I almost took early retirement last year because of the constant pain. However, the 7-Step Treatment Program has changed my life, and I've told my co-workers that I may never retire! I believe the twice-daily moist heat and stretching exercises have helped the most for the fibromyalgia and osteoarthritis pain, along with de-stressing, so I don't tense my neck or shoulders while sitting at the computer station."

- Donna, age forty-one, with all-over muscle pain and rheumatoid arthritis, said, "Before I started the 7-Step Treatment Program I felt like giving up on life. I was resigned to spending the second half of my life on the 'sidelines,' while my family and friends enjoyed their activities. Using this plan, I worked with my doctor to find the right combination of medications to resolve my pain. Then, using the twice-daily moist heat, stretching and resistance exercises, and lifestyle changes, I began to feel like my old (pain-free) self again. I take every step in the program very seriously as I don't ever want to feel relegated to my home because of chronic pain."

From Patient to Person

By now, you may be wondering if the 7-Step Treatment Program can help you to reclaim your pain-free, active life. There is only one way to find out: read the book, and start the program right now. Make a commitment to stick with the program for at least six weeks. If you can do that, I know that you'll change fibromyalgia from something disabling to a problem that is completely manageable. With the 7-Step Treatment Program, you can learn to identify and then treat each symptom effectively, and start to do the activities you enjoy in reasonable comfort without being overly medicated or feeling debilitating pain and stiffness.

You deserve to know that the high anxiety that accompanies fibromyalgia can make you feel broken, especially when you haven't got time for the pain, fatigue, and immobility. However, in the midst of the brokenness that you feel, I know that you can become a *whole person* again as you learn to conquer this disease instead of conceding to it.

Now let's get started.

1

WHAT IS FIBROMYALGIA?

"Aching, stabbing, and sometimes even burning." That's how forty-one-year-old Kelly, an FMS survivor, described the unending deep muscle pain in her neck, shoulders, and lower back. "The pain greets me the moment I get up, stays with me all throughout the day, and is still there when I crawl into bed at night."

"I've tried every medication—from aspirin to strong narcotics—and nothing works permanently to end the pain. On the other hand, if it does stop the pain, I usually suffer with horrible drug side effects like burning indigestion or nausea. On days when I have to keep up with my three children—driving carpools, packing lunches, and ironing school uniforms—my pain intensifies. Some days I think I cannot walk one more step or pick up my toddler because my back aches and my muscles throb. The sad part is I ignore my own personal needs just to make sure my family is cared for."

Over a period of two years, Kelly had been to three different doctors, trying to get an accurate diagnosis and treatment for the interminable pain, fatigue, and depression. When I finally saw her, she had lost twelve pounds because of the escalating stress and fear of what might lie ahead for her and her family, if these symptoms worsened. "I lie awake at night, wondering how

I will raise my kids, if my pain exacerbates. Sometimes I worry that my husband will leave me and the kids and seek a relationship with a healthy woman."

After running a few tests to eliminate other problems, I explained to Kelly that she had fibromyalgia, an arthritis-related syndrome. I convinced Kelly that if she stayed committed to the 7-Step Treatment Program, she would have reduced pain, better sleep, and more energy than she'd had in years. Kelly did just that, even though she had to try three different medications before finding the one that completely stopped her pain. She now rides bikes with her kids after school and uses meditation and other mind/body exercises to de-stress when she starts to feel overwhelmed with life's commitments. Kelly still has fibromyalgia. However, she has now learned how to take care of herself with a multifaceted treatment program.

If you've been diagnosed with fibromyalgia, I know that you identify with the deep muscle pain, difficulty maintaining restful sleep, unending fatigue, and even feelings of despair and depression of this condition. For those with FMS, these symptoms are chronic and severe, lasting for months and years and causing poor quality of life—damaging jobs, families, and personal lives. Nevertheless, I'm going to share with you new hope and help!

Rebecca came to our clinic because of widespread pain that she described as "stabbing and throbbing" from her shoulders and the back of her neck to her legs. This forty-seven-year-old woman worked full-time as a data processor, but in the past few months she had been unable to sit at the computer for any length of time due to the pain.

"I wake up every day with stabbing pain and think that maybe it will go away," she said. "When I get to work and sit at the computer, the pain worsens and often feels piercing, like a knife is in my muscle. I feel tired all the time and can't cook dinner for my family. If anyone touches me, I cringe because of the tenderness. Because of the exhaustion, I'm in bed by 7:30 P.M. each night, yet I never feel rested. What is wrong with me?"

After a careful examination and evaluation of the symptoms, this middle-aged woman was diagnosed with fibromyalgia. Coined in 1976, the term *fibromyalgia* describes the basic symptoms of constant muscle pain, tenderness, fatigue, and tender points. As Rebecca experienced, fibromyalgia causes widespread pain—in the back, neck, arms, and legs—with many tender or trigger points that are very painful when touched.

Fibromyalgia—with its deep muscle pain, disturbed sleep, and feelings of depression—affects more than 10 million Americans, with 90 percent being women. There are new estimates that as many as 8 percent of *all* women are affected by fibromyalgia. This may bring some comfort to the millions of women who thought the symptoms of fatigue, aching muscles, and low-grade depression were "mental" in nature.

Sophisticated research has shown that the syndrome can start in childhood or teenage years, especially with girls, and gradually worsens with age. Some recent studies show that because of the common symptoms, the disease may be vastly underdiagnosed in older adults, who often accept the unexplained pain in their bodies as another sign of aging. It is important to know up front that fibromyalgia is *not* a sign of aging!

Patients tell of going from doctor to doctor with symptoms of fatigue, which are present even on arising. They may have specific *tender points* on the body that hurt to the touch, or they may have pain all over. Forty-one-year-old Janis told of hurting everywhere on her body; even sitting in a straight-back chair brought tears to her eyes. Sarah, a young mother of two, felt throbbing pain all over her body as well as disturbances in deep-level, restful sleep, accompanied by feelings of sadness or depression. Mike felt a piercing pain in his neck and shoulders, accompanied by sluggishness, that came on suddenly after a car accident. While these patients had different manifestations of pain and fatigue, the symptoms were all the result of fibromyalgia.

A Common but Misunderstood Disease

Even though this has been a commonly misdiagnosed and mis-
understood syndrome, fibromyalgia is the most common arthritis-
related disease next to osteoarthritis. The consensus document
on fibromyalgia from the Second World Conference on Myofascial Pain and Fibromyalgia in 1992 reported that fibromyalgia
may be the most common cause of widespread musculoskeletal
pain.

Fibromyalgia was first described in medical documents more
than 150 years ago, yet even as recently as ten years ago, this
problem was rarely discussed in the medical community. Those
who don't understand it may not recognize that it exists. One
middle-aged woman recently brought her entire family in to our
clinic to talk about FMS. "Because I look healthy, they think I
overexaggerate my symptoms," she explained. "Please tell them
that I'm not making this up."

One must wonder how treatment can begin if the problem is
not recognized. For most people, it is common for the symptoms to drag on for months or years before a proper diagnosis is
made. In fact, for most patients, the average amount of time to
pass before diagnosis is made is *four to five years.* Imagine living
half a decade with debilitating symptoms and being told by family, friends, and your physician that the pain and fatigue are in
your head!

Thousands of patients each year tell of going from doctor to
doctor with symptoms of crippling fatigue and constant muscle
and joint pain all over their body. "Before I was diagnosed with
fibromyalgia, I was told by two doctors that nothing was wrong
with me," Vicky said, "and another suggested that my pain was
psychological."

While more and more people are receiving the proper diagnosis of fibromyalgia from physicians who understand this rheumatic disease, there are estimates that thousands of people are
still living with undiagnosed and untreated symptoms.

If you have been diagnosed with fibromyalgia or if you have the described symptoms and believe that this might be the problem, you have probably heard one or more of the following statements from friends and family members:

"It's all in your head."
"If you would relax more, you could sleep at night."
"Maybe you're too focused on yourself; get out and get busy."
"If you would exercise more, you wouldn't feel that muscle pain."
"Get a job. It will make you feel less depressed."
"You look healthy to me. Maybe you just want sympathy."
"You just don't want to feel good. Why do you always crave attention?"
"Slow down. Your life is so busy, it is making you crazy."
"Your life is wonderful, so don't be depressed."
"If the doctor says it's in your head, it must be true."
"If the lab tests do not show anything, you aren't sick."
"You act like this is the end of the world; lighten up."

After suffering with endless pain and chronic fatigue day after day, month after month, you may even begin to believe that you are fabricating the symptoms or that the problem really is in your mind. But this disease is very real.

Lydia, a forty-two-year-old lab technician and mother of two, was faced with early retirement due to the fatigue and even had to take catnaps throughout her workday to keep going. Lydia told of feeling widespread aching and stabbing pain in her muscles and joints, which greatly affected her ability to work and care for her family. She lived with these symptoms for four years and was evaluated by six doctors but did not receive a correct diagnosis.

When she came to our clinic, she felt tired, achy, and mildly depressed. But more important, Lydia was angry that no one could tell her what was happening to her body. "I guess because my symptoms and feelings come and go, the doctors thought that I was overworked or depressed," she said. "The antidepressant one doctor prescribed helped me sleep, but I still didn't feel rested in the morning, and I continued to hurt all over."

Darlene came to our clinic complaining of searing pain in her back, neck, and chest, along with throbbing headaches that occurred almost daily. This forty-five-year-old legal secretary and single mother of three had very specific *tender points* on the body that were painful to touch, along with regular disturbances in deep-level or restful sleep at night. Her main concern was the stiffness throughout her body on arising in the morning. "I have to work, but after walking up the stairs to my office, the pain is unbearable," she said.

Darlene's excruciating pain was worsened by any stress, a symptom that is quite common. She said that when the disease was active, her concentration at work was gravely affected, and she felt more irritable, even depressed. Another patient, forty-year-old Nina, had deep muscle pain in the abdomen along with dramatic changes in her bowel habits, ranging from constipation to diarrhea.

Darlene and Nina had frequency in urination with a sensation of an immediate urge to urinate; and both women complained of painful menstrual cramps, which are quite common in women with fibromyalgia. Nina had a pale discoloration of the fingers on cold exposure, such as holding a cold glass or putting a hand in the refrigerator.

Symptoms Come and Go

Peter, a middle-aged gentleman, came to see me about his symptoms, which had been ongoing for several months. He seemed a bit nervous during our conversation, and finally admitted that on the day of his evaluation, he was symptom-free. "I don't understand it," Peter said. "The last few days, I didn't ache at all, and last night I slept for the first time without tossing and turning."

Peter's case is not unusual. In fibromyalgia, the symptoms may come and go; therefore, it may be difficult to get proper diagnosis. If the physician does not understand the complexity of the disease, a patient may be sent away without any help or hope for treatment. In fact, studies show that *thousands* of patients each year tell of going from doctor to doctor with constant pain all over their body along with feelings of fatigue. Many are told that there is nothing wrong or that the problem is psychological.

Today we know differently. We know that fibromyalgia is a complex disorder characterized by *chronic* (meaning three months or longer) widespread pain, decreased pain threshold or tender points, and incapacitating fatigue. Women are ten times more likely to get the disease than men. While there is no specific laboratory test or abnormal X ray finding for diagnosis, the symptoms of the disease can be successfully treated once a proper diagnosis is made.

The Causes of Fibromyalgia

To see how the 7-Step Treatment Program can halt or even reverse fibromyalgia, you need to first understand what causes this nonspecific yet common syndrome. Once we understand the cause, scientists can find the exact tests to make an accurate diagnosis and then formulate specific treatments that target the root of the problem.

MALFUNCTION OF PAIN PROCESSING?
While there is no known cause of FMS, we do know that FMS is not all in patients' heads. Some investigators indicate that fibromyalgia symptoms may be the product of malfunctioning pain processing in the spinal cord, resulting in a central nervous system that "remembers" pain feelings for a longer time than usual. As a rule, pain subsides between stimuli. Nevertheless, with fibromyalgia, the pain memory appears to linger so that each succeeding stimulus results in greater pain feelings.

An enlightening brain-scan study published in the May 2002 issue of *Arthritis and Rheumatism* confirms that those with fibromyalgia feel pain that is severe, when compared with healthy people. To correlate pain sensation with views of brain signals, study investigators at Georgetown University Medical Center and the National Institutes of Health used a fast form of MRI (called functional MRI or functional magnetic resonance imaging) to test sixteen fibromyalgia patients and sixteen healthy patients. In the study, subjects had their brains scanned for more than ten minutes while a small device rapidly applied pressure to the base of their thumbnail. The pressure varied throughout the test period, but it was the same for each person.

During the test, researchers were able to capture the neurobiology of fibromyalgia's tenderness, which is characteristic of the set of symptoms, as the same mild pressure produced measurable brain responses in the FMS patients. This pressure had to be doubled to cause pain in the healthy subjects, causing researchers to conclude that FMS patients did have enhanced response to pain.

HYPERSENSITIVE TO PAIN?

Through numerous clinical studies, researchers have found that in people who suffer with chronic pain, the spinal cord becomes overloaded with input. This may make it oversensitive to any messages sent its way and causes the spinal cord to overreact to or amplify any response. When your body reacts hypersensitively in this way to pain, even a gentle breeze touching your skin will make you hurt. Recently scientists have concluded that fibromyalgia patients often feel higher sensitivity to pain over their entire body. This has led to the idea that with FMS, the body's overall pain threshold may be dramatically lower than usual.

GENETIC TENDENCY OR ELEVATED SUBSTANCE P LEVELS?

Some researchers think fibromyalgia may be the result of a genetic tendency; therefore, it may be passed on from generation to generation. When a person who has this tendency is exposed to certain emotional or physical stressors (like an illness or life crisis), there is a change in the body's response to stress. This can result in a higher sensitivity of the entire body to pain. Scientists theorize that one of these body changes is a low level of a hormone, CRH (corticotropin-releasing hormone), resulting in higher sensitivity to pain and more fatigue, including the fatigue experienced after exercise. Still other researchers have recently concluded that those with fibromyalgia have significantly less blood flow to the parts of the brain that deal with pain. In studies where fibromyalgia patients were compared to healthy people, those with FMS were found to have twice the level of a brain chemical called *substance P,* a neuropeptide involved in pain signals. This chemical helps nervous system cells send messages to each other about painful stimuli. It is thought that when substance P levels are elevated in the body, they may produce higher levels of pain.

LINKED TO STRESS?

Researchers indicate that fibromyalgia is linked to stress or other emotional illness. On the other hand, some findings show that psychological stress in the fibromyalgia patient is often high before the disease begins. No matter which is true, there is no denying that chronic pain *is* emotional, affecting every part of your being—your mind, body, and emotions. If your chronic muscle pain or overall body aches have lasted for months, you may have forgotten what it was like to be happy, carefree, and optimistic—even though you were a positive person before your symptoms started. Chronic pain slowly takes away your life; it interferes with your sleep, your ability to be physically active, your relationships, and your productivity on the job and at home. Is it any wonder that fibromyalgia patients tell of having high stress levels and some simply want to give up on life? There *is* a better way!

TRAUMA TO THE NERVOUS SYSTEM?

Some researchers indicate that FMS may be caused by bio-chemical changes in the body, for example, accidents, injuries, or illnesses. Other studies reveal that the disease may result from sudden trauma to the central nervous system.

A RESULT OF MENOPAUSE?

"Since I went through menopause, my symptoms have quadru-pled," Lois, a fifty-four-year-old retired teacher who was diag-nosed three years ago, said. "I had to quit teaching kindergarten because the pain in my shoulders and neck kept me from keep-ing up with my kids, and I felt so tired each day."

Some researchers have suggested that the loss of the female hormone *estrogen,* which happens at menopause, may trigger this disease. Hosts of experiments are being done to see if loss of estrogen does, in fact, stimulate this disease; it is true that fibromyalgia commonly occurs between the ages of forty and fifty-five, or around the time of menopause.

DUE TO AGING?

"Maybe fibromyalgia is similar to aging," Nancy surmised. "All these symptoms came on at midlife, and I have heard that all things fall apart after age forty."

The truth is that even though the disease occurs more fre-quently after the age of forty, there is no specific evidence that fibromyalgia is a problem of aging. It is also well known to occur in teenagers and gradually worsen over time. Furthermore, it does not continue to increase in much older people (seventy to eighty years old).

CONNECTED TO SEROTONIN?

Clearly, some research indicates that this hypersensitivity to pain may in part be from low levels of *serotonin,* a naturally occurring neurotransmitter in the body. (Neurotransmitters are

brain chemicals that send specific messages from one bra
to another.) Lower levels of serotonin cause a lower pain thi
old and disordered sleep. The result may be the chronic wid
spread pain of fibromyalgia. Some interesting studies revea
that women have approximately seven times less serotonin in
the brain, which may explain why FMS is more prevalent in
women than in men. Abnormal transport of serum *tryptophan*
(a precursor for serotonin) has also been described in clinical
findings, as well as deficiencies in *magnesium*.

FOR WOMEN ONLY?

Although I see men with fibromyalgia, the majority of sufferers
are women. In fact, fibromyalgia is thought to be the most common cause of generalized musculoskeletal pain in women
between the ages of twenty and fifty-five. We know that women
are more susceptible to pain, whether from hormones, the
lower serotonin levels, or just the way they are wired. For
instance, women are two to three times more likely to have
migraine headaches than men, and more women have
osteoarthritis and rheumatoid arthritis than their male counter-
parts. In a revealing 1999 Gallup Survey, investigators reported
that 46 percent of women interviewed had daily pain compared
to 37 percent of men, 17 percent of women had frequent
headaches, 24 percent had backaches, 20 percent had arthritis,
and one out of four women had aching feet. While we are
unsure as to the reason for a woman's increased susceptibility to
pain, we do know that it mandates different treatment than a
man's pain.

VITAMIN DEFICIENCY?

While linking fibromyalgia to a vitamin deficiency is still speculation, some new studies make this possible connection. Investigators presenting research at the American Association for the
Advancement of Science (2002) said that some people with

e a chronic vitamin D deficiency. These
that getting out in the sun for just five to
e times a week is enough to boost your
her this will help calm your symptoms
at vitamin D is a crucial nutrient to
rong and prevent osteoporosis, the thinning
you have dark skin, you will need ten to twenty
the length of sun that light-skinned people need to keep
your body's vitamin D supplies adequate.

AFTER INJURY OR AS A RESULT OF LYME DISEASE?

Fibromyalgia often occurs following an injury, even one that
may be mild, or after a bout with the flu. Some patients diagnosed with Lyme disease, which can cause muscle and joint
pain, along with other problems, and is spread through the bite
of a tick, were found to have fibromyalgia as their main problem. No specific evidence was found that Lyme disease caused
fibromyalgia in those patients.

POOR PHYSICAL CONDITIONING
OR AS A RESULT OF DEPRESSION?

Some studies support the theory that people who are unfit are
more likely to get fibromyalgia. Speculation is that stress and
poor physical conditioning may both be major factors in the
cause of the disease.

Other studies have shown that because fibromyalgia is
accompanied by low-grade depression, there may be a link
between these two illnesses. Some researchers feel that depression leads to changes in the chemistry of the brain or that abnormalities of the sympathetic nervous system result in the release
of substances that cause more sensitivity to pain, resulting in
fibromyalgia.

UNKNOWN CAUSES?

Although there are many theories on what causes fibromyalgia, the truth remains unknown. For many years doctors thought that the disease was caused by a disorder of the muscles or that it was a psychological problem. Some researchers believe that this mysterious syndrome has a genetic disposition, as it can run in families. The most recent research suggests that the muscles themselves are not the source of the pain, but rather that the pain is a response to changes in the brain. All of these explanations remain unproven, but research is continuing.

No single theory seems to explain all of the problems in fibromyalgia. Whatever the cause, the vicious cycle of pain and disturbed sleep leads to less activity, greater depression, and more pain. This pain cycle can incapacitate the sufferer for months and possibly years unless the proper treatment is administered to control the symptoms. While there is no cure, the symptoms *can* be successfully treated.

The Feelings of Fibromyalgia

Because fibromyalgia can cause signs and feelings similar to osteoarthritis, bursitis, and tendinitis, some specialists include it in the group of arthritis and related disorders. But unlike the bursitis or tendinitis, which is usually localized to a single area, the feelings of pain and stiffness associated with fibromyalgia are widespread. In fact, if there are not many areas involved, then it does not fit the typical picture of fibromyalgia. If a joint is warm or swollen or does not move properly, then there is probably another problem present, such as another form of arthritis or an injury.

For some patients, fibromyalgia's symptoms are not always constant—the pain comes and goes. Unlike some severe forms of arthritis that cause crippling, most fibromyalgia patients are able to get through the day, though they constantly feel tired and achy.

COMMON SYMPTOMS OF FIBROMYALGIA

Pain

Fatigue

Morning stiffness

Trigger points

Sleep problems

Anxiety

Difficulty in concentration

Depression

Swelling, numbness, and tingling in hands, arms, feet, and
   legs

Headaches

Irritable bowel syndrome (abdominal pain, constipation,
   diarrhea)

Urinary symptoms (burning, frequency)

Painful menstrual cramps

Discoloration of hands and feet (Raynaud's phenomenon)

Restless legs syndrome

Dryness in mouth, nose, and eyes

PAIN: THE MOST COMMON SYMPTOM

Pain plays a significant role in the diagnosis of fibromyalgia and
is usually the major complaint that signals a visit to the doctor.
This widespread pain is characteristic of more than 97 percent
of patients. Unlike the pain of osteoarthritis, bursitis, or tendinitis, which is usually relegated to a specific joint or area, this pain
can be felt over the entire body and is deep, sharp, dull, throbbing, or aching. There may also be accompanying pain in the
joints, such as the shoulders, hips, back, and neck. Joint pain can
also come from the hands, wrists, elbows, knees, ankles, and
feet. However, even more common is pain felt in the muscles,
tendons, and ligaments around the joints.

Peggy was diagnosed strictly from the pain she was experiencing. "I live day and night with a sharp, throbbing pain in the
muscles in my neck and shoulders, yet I have not experienced

the fatigue that usually accompanies this. The pain becomes especially intense after exercise or housework, especially when I do chores such as sweeping, mopping, vacuuming, or washing windows. The pain becomes so unbearable that sometimes prescription pain medications do not touch it."

Other patients who tell of feeling pain in the back, neck, and head complain also of frequent headaches. Many times these pains are from the muscles and other soft tissues around the back and neck, not from fibromyalgia.

I often see patients who have had a back injury, such as a ruptured disc in the lower part of the spine (lumbar spine). These patients have had surgery on the lower back or neck for treatment of the injury. After a neck or back injury, which may result in bed rest and loss of activity, many patients develop symptoms of fibromyalgia for reasons that are unknown.

RELENTLESS FATIGUE IS CRIPPLING

Next to pain and the tender trigger points, fatigue is a major complaint. We *all* know what it feels like to be tired. However, because we are each different, we may have dissimilar ideas of the meaning of *fatigue*. What is fatigue to you may not be the same for me or someone else. Fatigue in fibromyalgia refers to a lingering tiredness that is constant and limiting. For example, patients complain of being tired even when they should feel rested and have had enough sleep. Some patients admit to feeling sleepy, but much more common is a feeling of exhaustion without feeling drowsy. Some compare it to having the flu or to the feeling after working very long hours and missing a lot of sleep.

Just as the cause of fibromyalgia is not known, the exact cause of the fatigue is not known. Sleep disturbances, common in the large majority of patients, may help create a constant state of fatigue. In fact, hosts of experiments have shown that many of fibromyalgia's symptoms can actually be created in otherwise healthy people if their sleep is disturbed. Fatigue is so bothersome in many patients that they often say, "Please get rid of the fatigue, and I'll put up with the pain."

THE FATIGUE OF FIBROMYALGIA
Fatigued on arising in the morning
Fatigued after mild activity, such as grocery shopping or cooking dinner
Too fatigued to start a standard project, such as folding clothes or ironing
Too fatigued to exercise
Even more fatigued after exercise
Too fatigued for sex
Too fatigued to function adequately at work

MORNING STIFFNESS AFFECTS MOST PATIENTS
More than 75 percent of fibromyalgia patients feel stiffness in the morning on arising. This stiffness creates a feeling of the need to loosen up after getting out of bed before usual activities can begin, and the stiffness is extensive, going throughout the muscles and joints of the back, arms, and legs. In some patients, the morning stiffness may last only a few minutes, but it is usually very noticeable for more than fifteen or twenty minutes each day. Other patients report that the stiffness lasts for hours or even seems to be present all day. Most people feel stiff when they wake up, but this type of stiffness is very different than minor aching. In fact, this is the same feeling of stiffness in the morning that happens in many types of arthritis, especially rheumatoid arthritis.

TRIGGER POINTS
Many influences are at work in fibromyalgia. Patients like Peggy feel sharp, throbbing muscle pain. But accompanying this deep muscle soreness are painful *trigger points,* or localized areas of tenderness around joints (not joints themselves) that hurt when

pressed with a finger. These can be deep areas of pain but are often superficial areas seemingly under the surface of the skin, such as over the elbow or shoulder.

The cause of these trigger points is not known. Even though it would seem that these areas should be inflamed, no particular signs of inflammation have been found by researchers when the tissues are examined. The locations of the trigger points are not random; they are in predictable places on the body (see page 58).

SLEEP PROBLEMS

Most people with fibromyalgia syndrome are really bothered by sleep problems. The most common complaint is simply not having restful sleep, which is usually related to frequent "awakenings." During these awakenings, you may not notice being fully awake, but you are aroused enough to feel unrefreshed the next morning. While some researchers hold strongly to the belief that FMS may be due to nonrestorative deep sleep, sleep disorder is not thought to be the only cause of fibromyalgia.

The exact cause of the sleep disorder is not known, but scientists have discovered abnormal amounts of *alpha activity* on an electroencephalogram taken of FMS patients. (The electroencephalogram is a test done during a sleep study or polysomnography, which is discussed in chapter 8.) Alpha activity in the brain is associated with feelings of serenity and calmness, whereas beta activity is related to alertness.

It may be that disordered sleep leads to lower levels of serotonin, common in those with FMS, resulting in increased pain sensitivity. Researchers have demonstrated what amounts to "lower pain threshold" induced by sleep deprivation in healthy volunteers, which is also associated with an abnormal brain wave pattern.

Even though poor sleep doesn't create the fibromyalgia, it can make you feel exhausted upon awakening. This results in more pain, more sleep problems, and more fatigue. Interestingly, FMS-like symptoms have been induced in normal volunteers who were deprived of sleep—except in those who regularly exercised. The reason for this is that exercise increases the time you spend in deep sleep and has been found to be an excellent therapy for FMS patients. Some ways you can begin an exercise program are discussed in chapter 5.

Some people may have coexisting sleep disorders, in addition to fibromyalgia. For instance, restless legs syndrome is a condition many fibromyalgia sufferers complain of that is characterized by discomfort of the legs, especially below the knee, mainly at night. The feeling is most commonly described as the need to move the legs to try to make them comfortable. Restless legs syndrome often interrupts sleep as the person tries to find the most comfortable position for rest. As with other symptoms, restless legs syndrome can be found with other medical problems and has no effective treatment.

Sleep apnea is another concomitant sleep problem with fibromyalgia. In fact, in one study, sleep apnea was found in 40 percent of males with fibromyalgia. With this potentially life-threatening problem, a person stops breathing for periods called apneas, which are caused by obstruction of the upper airway at the level of the uvula or base of the tongue. Apneas may be interrupted by brief arousals that do not awaken you completely; in fact, you may not even realize you were disturbed during sleep. Those with obstructive sleep apnea may also have other very serious symptoms after what they thought was a good night's sleep as the arousals disturb or even ruin the normally refreshing nature of sleep. Low oxygen levels, which result when the blockages prevent air from getting to the lungs, also affect brain and heart function. In these cases, going to a sleep disorder clinic for polysomnography (a sleep study done in a special laboratory) can help in making the diagnosis and treating the symptoms.

COMMON SYMPTOMS OF OBSTRUCTIVE SLEEP APNEA (OSA)

- morning headaches
- high blood pressure
- dry mouth
- sore throat upon awakening
- depression
- concentration problems
- memory failure
- impotence
- excessive daytime sleepiness
- restless sleep (increased movements)
- choking sensations
- frequent awakenings
- irregular heart rhythm

COMMON SLEEP-RELATED SYMPTOMS WITH FMS

- I have frequent headaches in the morning upon getting out of bed.
- I feel muscle aches and pains throughout my body most of the time.
- I feel fatigue or tiredness that does not go away even after several large cups of strongly caffeinated coffee.
- I feel in a low mood that does not lift even as I get on with my daily activities.
- I have felt depressed enough to get antidepressants from my doctor.
- I feel irritable, impatient, and have mood swings.
- I often have difficulty being with a large group, as it feels overwhelming.
- I have trouble learning new information or grasping new ideas.
- I am unable to recall useful information and feel "foggy" sometimes.

DEPRESSION DISRUPTS DAILY ACTIVITIES

Depression (technically termed by psychologists and psychiatrists as either "major depression," in more severe cases, or "adjustment disorder with depressed mood," in less severe cases) is a very common response to chronic pain. However, in fibromyalgia, depression is one of the key markers. While not all FMS patients have depression, findings show that 25 percent of patients with fibromyalgia have current major depression; 50 percent have a life history of depression. Stress from the chronic pain and fatigue can cause anxiety, disordered sleep, less activity, and withdrawal—all of which can lead to depression.

Depression is primarily a disorder of mood, characterized by profound sadness, discouragement, and hopelessness. When a chronic illness such as fibromyalgia is the cause, the onset tends to be gradual. Perhaps you've experienced how living each day with chronic pain and fatigue weighs heavier than the last. Many patients complain of a loss of energy, general fatigue, or insomnia, combined with feelings of worthlessness ("My body has failed me!") and guilt ("What have I done to deserve this?"). Seeking treatment for the chronic body aches and muscle pain may produce an initial boost in mood ("Maybe this will be the answer!"). Still, this rise often sets you up for even greater disappointment when your doctor says, "There is no cure for fibromyalgia." Every new medication—usually more costly than the last—produces renewed optimism. Every failed attempt to put a stop to this ruthless syndrome brings you crashing back to earth—and reality. In addition, the pain-relieving drugs may well exacerbate mood disturbances, increasing your anxiety and irritability. Finally, among those men and women who suffer with relentless pain and have to give up their careers, depression may turn to grief. Periods of denial, bargaining, and anger will intermingle with depression until, hopefully, a state of acceptance establishes itself, and you move forward to seek effective treatment and gain relief of your symptoms.

"FIBRO FOG" INTERFERES WITH CONCENTRATION AND JOB PERFORMANCE

Fibromyalgia patients often tell of great difficulty keeping their attention concentrated on their work or other activities. Some complain of memory problems, especially for events that happened recently, along with general confusion and forgetfulness at times. The hazy mental feeling has been called "fibro fog," and it can interfere with daily activities and work. For some fibromyalgia patients, fibro fog is an overwhelming problem that makes them unable to work. The periods of lowered concentration and memory can result in loss of information, confusion, and lower function.

Researchers have found that a majority of fibromyalgia patients experience the problems of fibro fog with memory and mental clarity problems. Many experience problems with dissociation, which results in a loss of mental connection from complete awareness of everyday events. Some experts believe that dissociation might help explain some of the problems of fibro fog, as mild dissociation can be the result of poor sleep or medications. While these problems are difficult to measure and may not show up as an abnormality on tests given to fibromyalgia patients, they are still very real. If the tests are negative, it does add to the frustration of fibromyalgia patients.

EACH DAY INCREASES ANXIETY

Another psychological feeling with fibromyalgia is anxiety. After living with chronic muscle pain and overall body aches for months, you may become obsessed with how you feel each day, noticing every new feeling or symptom. Complaints of general nervousness and irritability, excessive worry, and sleep problems are common. Anxiety may also take the form of specific phobias (such as fear of being alone, fear of driving, or fear of exercise). Alternatively, you may find yourself completely angry or bitter toward your doctor, your family, or even life in general.

The cost of anxiety and depression is high as it greatly interferes with your activities at work and at home. The symptoms can be successfully treated with a combination of medication and therapy, so it's important to discuss these feelings openly with your doctor.

SWELLING AND TINGLING HANDS CAN BE A PROBLEM

While the cause is not known, many patients have a feeling of swelling in the hands, arms, feet, or legs. The feeling may be especially bothersome upon arising, especially in combination with morning stiffness, yet does not appear to limit activity.

Numbness or tingling sensations in the hands, arms, or legs are also reported by more than half of all fibromyalgia patients. The medical term for these feelings is *paresthesia*. The sensations happen irregularly and usually last a few minutes, though they can be constant. Although these sensations may be bothersome, they are not severely limiting.

CHRONIC HEADACHES ARE PART OF THE DISEASE

More than half of all fibromyalgia patients suffer from chronic headaches. While 50 to 75 percent of patients suffer with migraine headaches, many patients complain of *tension-type* or *muscle contraction headaches* caused by tightness in and contraction of the muscles of the neck. The FMS headache feels like a dull pain in the forehead or back of the head, or both, with tightness or pressure in or around the head. The pain may extend over the top of your head to the front near your eyebrows. Some patients describe the headache as feeling like you're wearing a metal cap that's several sizes too small, and it keeps getting smaller as it relentlessly squeezes your head. You may also have soreness in the tender trigger points in the back of your head and the neck. Your jaws may also hurt if there is tightness of the muscles in these areas. It's important to remember that headaches can be caused by other medical problems, which should be properly diagnosed and treated by your doctor.

IRRITABLE BOWEL SYNDROME AFFECTS SUFFERERS

Irritable bowel syndrome (IBS) is a condition characterized by abdominal cramps and pain, along with periods of diarrhea alternating with bouts of constipation. About one-third of fibromyalgia patients suffer from IBS. Complaints can include excessive gas and bloating along with the irritable bowel syndrome.

URINARY FREQUENCY CAN OCCUR

A feeling of the urge to urinate, which is a condition called *urinary urgency,* painful or frequent urination, and incontinence have been found in about 25 percent of fibromyalgia patients. Since these problems can also be caused by other bladder and kidney diseases, it is important to check with your doctor to be sure no other specific problems are present.

PAINFUL MENSTRUAL CRAMPS AFFECT FEMALE PATIENTS

Painful menstrual cramps are found in 30 to 40 percent of women with fibromyalgia. Most women who suffer with cramps also experience aching in the upper thighs, along with lower back pain, bloating and abdominal distension, nausea, diarrhea, and fatigue, among other symptoms. These cramps, categorized as "primary dysmenorrhea," are usually caused by the elevated production of prostaglandins, hormones produced by the uterus that cause it to contract. When you have strong uterine contractions, the blood supply to the uterus is momentarily shut down, depriving the uterine muscle of oxygen and setting up the cycle of menstrual contractions and pain. There are many serious problems such as a uterine fibroid tumor, endometriosis, or pelvic infection that can cause menstrual cramps, so be sure to check with your doctor to make sure no other treatment is needed.

Chronic pelvic pain is another common complaint of this condition, particularly from women of childbearing age. This pain could be gynecological in nature, or it may stem from irritable bowel syndrome (IBS), interstitial cystitis (IC), or pelvic floor myofascial syndrome. You may experience this continuous or intermittent pelvic pain for months with no known cause or cure.

DISCOLORATION OF EXTREMITIES

Some patients notice that their fingers or, though less commonly, their toes become pale, cold, or turn blue when exposed to cold—even such a small exposure as holding a cold glass. The pale or blue changes may last for a few minutes and can be accompanied by pain. When the hands or feet are warmed, they return to normal.

This problem is called *Raynaud's Phenomenon,* which affects up to 40 percent of those with fibromyalgia. While it can happen in otherwise normal persons and is also a characteristic of other medical problems, such as other types of arthritis, it is your doctor who can make sure no other medical problems are present. Sometimes, medications are needed to control this symptom.

DRYNESS IS A CONCERN

Dryness of the mouth, nose or eyes can happen in otherwise normal persons, but more than 25 percent of fibromyalgia patients have this symptom. Dryness occurs when glands do not produce the normal amounts or quality of tears to lubricate the eyes or saliva to lubricate the mouth. This problem is commonly associated with rheumatoid and other types of arthritis and is called *Sjögren's syndrome.* There is no single known cause.

Although dryness is mainly uncomfortable, the loss of normal lubrication for the eyes can increase the risk of infection. The loss of normal saliva and lubrication in the mouth increases the chance of tooth decay. See your ophthalmologist and/or dentist for treatment.

Factors That Worsen Symptoms

In many studies, patients report that weather changes greatly affect musculoskeletal symptoms. In fact, those with the highest weather sensitivity tend to have more functional impairment and psychological distress.

FMS can also worsen during times of great stress or after exercise. Conversely, the chronic pain can subside during less stressful times. Beverly, age thirty-seven, told of living with chronic pain for months. Then, during a two-week cruise to the Caribbean with her husband, she became almost pain-free.

"After a few days into the cruise, I started sleeping through the night without awakening, and I was able to sightsee without resting periodically for the muscle pain. I thought I was healed, except that it was short-lived.

"Almost one month after my vacation, the aches and pain started again, and this time it was worse than ever. Somehow, I know that lessening my stress helped me reduce symptoms."

FACTORS THAT CAN WORSEN FIBROMYALGIA SYMPTOMS
Anxiety and depression
Changes in weather (cold or humidity)
Fatigue
Injuries
Lack of sleep or restless sleep
Other illnesses
Periods of emotional stress
Physical exhaustion
Sedentary lifestyle (lack of exercise)

Fibromyalgia Increases Daily Stress

As sufferers live with the symptoms of fibromyalgia, they can become increasingly focused on their pain and sadness, which is very real. The many appointments with health care providers to try to find relief, combined with the cost of these attempts, add to the patient's frustration.

As time goes on, patients have trouble keeping a job because of their many absences. As income declines, there can be more financial stresses to be dealt with by the sufferer and family. These stresses, along with the constant fatigue, pain, and low-grade depression, can cause severe relationship problems in the family.

The longer the situation lasts, the more likely a patient will see signs of stress, including:

Constant tiredness
Difficulty concentrating
Increasing irritability
Withdrawal from other activities (especially enjoyable ones)
Change in appetite
Depression

Fibromyalgia is an intrapersonal experience—not just a diagnosis. This means the chronic deep muscle pain and other symptoms encompass everything about you—your feelings, emotions, attitude, as well as the pain you feel. Once you understand the many ways the syndrome manifests itself and the stress and other feelings that accompany the disease, you can begin steps to control your reaction (see chapters 6 and 7) and reclaim control of your life.

The Cost of Fibromyalgia

In addition to the human cost in suffering to the patient and family, the expenses associated with this disease can be devastating. Health care and medication costs can run to many thousands of dollars, not including the costs of specialized tests, counseling, or hospitalization.

After an extended course of treatment with little control of pain and more loss of activity, patients may be referred to a pain clinic. An inpatient pain clinic with a four-to-six-week treatment can be helpful, but this alone may cost $20,000 or more.

The good news is that large savings in health care costs are possible if the symptoms can be controlled. And the improvement in human costs could affect millions of people.

Take a Proactive Approach to Healing

The fact is, the outlook for people with fibromyalgia is remarkably better than ever before. Ongoing research and scientific trials are providing new information on the disease and how to treat the symptoms successfully. However, the first step in controlling these symptoms is understanding all you can about the disease, including the recommended modes of treatment and seeking a proper diagnosis, which is explained in chapter 3. Most patients feel a noticeable decrease in pain and fatigue and an increase in mobility and energy within a few months of starting treatment. This is exactly what happened to Helen, who has lived with this mysterious disease for two years.

This young attorney told of having throbbing muscle pain when she was in law school. "I was so stressed all the time from trying to compete in my class that I just assumed that the pain and tiredness I felt were caused by this," she told me. "But when I left law school and joined a large practice in town, I continued to have the same symptoms."

Helen lived with undiagnosed fibromyalgia and quietly suffered its life-stealing symptoms. When she was still in school, she worked her schedule around daily nap periods and avoided heavy activity or sports for fear of more pain and fatigue. Today she is a different person. She has learned that although the symptoms still wax and wane, she can actively tackle these symptoms with lifestyle changes that make a difference in how she feels each day.

Everyone Is Different

Remember, each person is different. The more specific the diagnosis of arthritis and rheumatic diseases, the more specific the treatment can be. This book cannot replace a proper medical diagnosis. It was written to help you become more informed about fibromyalgia so that you can knowledgeably seek a professional diagnosis from your doctor and begin treatment.

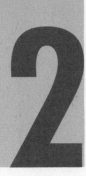

FIBROMYALGIA WITH OTHER PAIN-RELATED CONDITIONS

As you seek answers for the disabling pain, fatigue, and other fibromyalgia symptoms, it's important that your doctor determine which signs and symptoms are caused by fibromyalgia and which are not. While fibromyalgia can happen alone, many people are not aware that it can also occur with another arthritis, such as osteoarthritis, rheumatoid arthritis, or other types of arthritis. You might have FMS along with back pain from a previous injury or disc disease. Alternatively, you could have FMS and carpal tunnel syndrome or bursitis.

I know that when you have more than one health problem, it makes a painful condition even more confusing and frustrating. Yet, once your doctor determines the cause of your pain, he or she can prescribe an effective medical and lifestyle plan that will resolve all of the symptoms and let you return to an active life.

Dory, a thirty-seven-year-old real estate broker, was initially treated by her primary care doctor for fibromyalgia. Yet, after about four years, she started having increased pain and stiffness. When I evaluated Dory, she said her hands were stiff and swollen in the mornings on awakening, and she had trouble opening jars and using the computer because her fingers hurt. In addition, she had swelling in her feet that made wearing shoes and even walking much more painful.

After undergoing some tests, I diagnosed Dory with rheumatoid arthritis in addition to the fibromyalgia. When she began
specific treatment for both conditions, she noticed all-over
improvement in pain and stiffness. She became more comfortable at work, and her sleep and energy improved.

Just like fibromyalgia, rheumatoid arthritis is common in
young women and some of the symptoms are similar. For
instance, both ailments cause unending fatigue, as well as stiffness in the morning on arising. Therefore, it's not surprising that
it's often difficult to sort out the true causes of the problems.
Nevertheless, once an accurate diagnosis is made, each problem can be treated specifically and individually. In many cases,
controlling both problems helps to resolve the overall pain and
other symptoms.

After reading about some of the most common arthritis and
pain-related conditions that might cause confusion when you're
in constant pain, review the chart on page 51. It shows how different pain-related problems often mimic fibromyalgia's signs
and symptoms. Yet, each ailment has specialized treatment.

Fibromyalgia Classification

1. Fibromyalgia without any other underlying disease,
   such as osteoarthritis or other types of arthritis
2. Fibromyalgia along with another disease, such as
   osteoarthritis, rheumatoid arthritis, or systemic lupus
   erythematosus (SLE)

---

100 Different Types of Arthritis

With more than a hundred types of arthritis, even experienced
arthritis specialists can have trouble deciding which type of
arthritis you might have, much less separating your fibromyalgia
symptoms from another type of pain. Yet, the idea that all

arthritis is alike has led many people to use treatments that have little effect. Since each kind of arthritis may require a special type of treatment, a precise diagnosis is essential. Then you'll know what causes the pain, and you can take steps to relieve this properly and continue to be active. What works for someone else's arthritis or pain-related condition may not work for you. Therefore, I find it easier to understand if we divide arthritis into two main categories, as shown below. I will then discuss the most common types of arthritis within these two categories that often occur with fibromyalgia.

1. Osteoarthritis or "degenerative arthritis" are the wear-and-tear arthritis types;
2. Inflammatory types of arthritis are those in which the linings of joints become inflamed.

THE MOST COMMON TYPES OF ARTHRITIS

GROUP 1 **Osteoarthritis Group**	GROUP 2 **Inflammatory Arthritis Group**
Osteoarthritis	Rheumatoid arthritis
Fibromyalgia	Systemic lupus erythematosus
Bursitis	PMR (polymyalgia rheumatica)
Tendinitis	Gout
Carpal tunnel syndrome	Ankylosing Spondylitis
	Arthritis with psoriasis
	Many others

Osteoarthritis

When Nancy was referred to me by her primary care doctor, she literally ached all over. Even though she had been diagnosed with fibromyalgia and had started treatment, Nancy still complained of pain and stiffness in her knee and hip and was contemplating early retirement because she hurt all the time. This forty-seven-year-old high school principal was also about thirty pounds overweight, which contributed to her knee and hip pain.

After doing a physical examination and running a few tests, I explained to Nancy how osteoarthritis, the "wear and tear" type of arthritis, is a completely different problem from fibromyalgia, which causes deep muscle pain and overall body aches. While both are painful ailments, osteoarthritis is joint-specific and mandates different therapies to alleviate the joint pain and stiffness. Having both pain-related problems only intensified the aching and fatigue Nancy felt, making it difficult to be effective in her administrative responsibilities at the high school. Yet, once both diseases were treated, she would notice a significant difference in decreased pain, less fatigue, and greater energy.

WHAT IS OSTEOARTHRITIS?

Osteoarthritis is the most common type of arthritis and usually attacks men and women over fifty. Still, it can hit earlier, especially in the hands or in other key joints following an injury. For instance, the weekend athlete who injures a knee or an ankle playing tennis may develop osteoarthritis in the injured joint. Or if you were an avid dancer or runner during young adult years, you may get osteoarthritis in the knee or ankle sooner than others. In addition, if you've fallen and injured your back, you are a prime candidate for osteoarthritis in the lower spine.

Tagged the "wear-and-tear" type of arthritis, osteoarthritis is more common in women. In fact, while women account for about 65 percent of all arthritis cases, they account for 74 percent of osteoarthritis cases (15.3 million women). As I explain in my book *Stop Osteoarthritis Now: Halting the Baby Boomer's Disease* (Fireside, 1996), osteoarthritis commonly hits joints including those that bear weight such as the knees, hips, and the back. These joints may become intensely painful and swollen, making it difficult to be active.

SIGNS AND SYMPTOMS

In osteoarthritis, you will feel well except for the specific joints involved. You may notice a few minutes of stiffness on arising in the morning, along with some stiffness after sitting for a short period. Nevertheless, these symptoms are usually not as severe as in the inflammatory types of arthritis such as rheumatoid arthritis. There are no internal organ problems in osteoarthritis.

DIAGNOSIS AND TREATMENT

Your doctor can diagnose osteoarthritis after taking X rays and a few blood tests. Treatments include anti-inflammatory drugs, exercises, and in some cases injections of various medications into a joint or surgery to control pain.

RISK FACTORS FOR OSTEOARTHRITIS

Age (older than forty-five years)

Injury

Heavy, constant joint use

Athletics (wear and tear and injuries from athletics)

Overweight

Knee surgery

Abnormal joint positions

Changing forces (putting weight on one knee or hip)

Joint injury by other types of arthritis

Gender (between forty-five and fifty-five, the chance of OA is the same for men and women; after age fifty-five, OA is more common in women)

Lack of exercise (weak muscles giving no support to aging joints)

SYMPTOMS OF OSTEOARTHRITIS

Deep, aching pain in joint

Swelling of joint

Joint may be warm to touch

Morning stiffness

Stiffness after resting

Fatigue
Pain when walking
Difficulty gripping objects
Difficulty dressing or combing hair
Difficulty sitting or bending over

Bursitis and Tendinitis

When Jennifer's shoulder pain did not go away after almost one month, she called for an evaluation. This young mother of twins suffered with fibromyalgia, which had been diagnosed previously. Yet after the twins were born, she noticed her left shoulder aching and nothing would resolve the pain. She said the pain intensified at night, especially when she would roll over on her side. Because of the pain, she had lost hours of sleep and was finding it difficult to keep up with her active babies.

I examined Jennifer and found that she had bursitis in her shoulder, possibly the result of lifting and carrying her twins. With bursitis, the bursa, a sac through which a tendon or muscle moves, becomes inflamed and causes extreme pain. This can happen in the shoulder, hip, or other area.

Jennifer noticed that anytime she moved her arm or shoulder she had severe pain. This is typical of bursitis. You might have mild or even severe pain anytime there is movement of the joint or even pressure on the joint, and the pain can last for weeks to months. The most common sites for bursitis are the shoulders, hips, knees, elbows, or buttocks. Repetitive movements, such as painting, yard work, or even lifting a baby, can frequently trigger an attack of bursitis, especially if not done regularly.

Tendinitis happens when a tendon becomes inflamed, such as around the elbow (tennis elbow or golfer's elbow), and can make movement painful. This can cause severe pain, especially when the muscle is used. One of the most common types of tendinitis occurs at the elbow, where it is called *tennis elbow* because the movements in tennis can trigger an attack. Other common sites are the shoulder, Achilles tendon, and the heel.

Tendinitis can happen alone or along with true arthritis in the nearby joint. In some cases, tendinitis can progress to what we call a "frozen shoulder." When this happens the ligaments and tendons around the shoulder may progressively stiffen until the joint can barely move without pain.

Both of these conditions can happen along with fibromyalgia and can be treated effectively to control the pain. Local injections (see page 94) often give quick relief of bursitis and tendinitis.

Carpal Tunnel Syndrome

Thirty-four-year old Matthew, a technical writer, was confused when he continued to suffer with numbness and tingling in the fingers of both hands. He said his family doctor had told him it was associated with fibromyalgia syndrome. Yet, when the medications and other treatments he used over several months failed to resolve the pain, he came in for an evaluation.

WHAT IS CARPAL TUNNEL SYNDROME?

After doing a physical examination and taking Matthew's medical history, I ran a few tests and diagnosed him with carpal tunnel syndrome. Many times this condition is confused with fibromyalgia, which may also cause numbness and tingling in the hands. Carpal tunnel syndrome (CTS) is a condition in which the median nerve that travels down the arm into the hand becomes compressed as it passes through a narrow path or tunnel at the wrist. Overuse can cause the tissues in the area to swell, and this swelling compresses the median nerve, resulting in the symptoms of numbness and pain.

While carpal tunnel syndrome can occur at any age, it is more common in those who are middle-aged or older. It is also reported 1.7 times more often by working women than men. More women than men also experience musculoskeletal injuries to the hand, wrist, arm, and shoulder caused by child care responsibilities requiring lifting and bending. Younger people usually get CTS because of an injury or repetitive stress on the wrist. For instance, if you are a musician, typist, or, as in Matthew's case, work at a computer, you are at a greater risk of getting carpal tunnel syndrome.

SIGNS AND SYMPTOMS

The symptoms of CTS include pain, tingling, or numbness in the thumb and next three fingers with the exception of the little finger. You may also feel swelling in your fingers. Sometimes there may be pain that travels from the hand up the arm possibly to the elbow.

Matthew complained of pain, numbness, and tingling that worsened at night and while driving, holding the telephone, or using his computer keyboard. He said he'd wake up frequently at night with his hands asleep and have to shake them to try to regain feeling. Some patients tell of the pain worsening when they were warm and improving when they were cold.

DIAGNOSIS AND TREATMENT

Your doctor can diagnose CTS after a complete physical examination, specifically noting the type of pain you have and the exact places on your hand. Tests including an electrical nerve conduction test may be helpful in obtaining an accurate diagnosis. With CTS, X rays and blood tests are usually normal. Depending on the exact cause, treatment may include a nonsteroid anti-inflammatory drug (NSAIDs), along with a splint for your wrist, a local injection of cortisone to reduce the swelling around the nerve, or possibly a minor outpatient surgical procedure.

Rheumatoid Arthritis

Sharon had been a fibromyalgia patient for more than a decade, but was now concerned that her college-age daughter, Kaitlyn, was experiencing severe fatigue and pain, as well as swelling in her hands and knees.

When I saw Kaitlyn, she said she'd lost more than fifteen pounds in just three months but thought it was because of the stress of college life and poor eating habits. She also complained of feeling exhausted and wanting to sleep all the time. Even with twelve hours of sleep, she still felt tired and had no energy. Kaitlyn finally quit her part-time campus job and dropped one course, hoping to get through the semester so she could graduate on time.

After a physical examination and some laboratory tests, I diagnosed Kaitlyn with rheumatoid arthritis, along with fibromyalgia. I explained to the young woman that it was no wonder she felt so tired all the time and promised we could get control of both problems to decrease the pain and fatigue and give her back her active life.

WHAT IS RHEUMATOID ARTHRITIS?

Rheumatoid arthritis is an inflammatory arthritis that affects up to 10 million Americans. Like fibromyalgia, it is more common in women, particularly young women. With this inflammatory type of arthritis, you may feel pain, swelling, stiffness, and warmth around the joints. As your own immune cells and their products eat away at your cartilage, your bones will eventually erode, causing deformities and crippling. This is because the prostaglandins, which cause inflammation, trigger enzymes that cause pain and swelling, in turn triggering other enzymes that attack the cartilage and bones in the joints. There may be small areas of bones that become damaged and destroyed but over a few years, these changes can add up to joint deformity and limited use.

SIGNS AND SYMPTOMS

Rheumatoid arthritis comes on gradually with pain, stiffness, and swelling in some combination of hands, wrists, elbows, shoulders, knees, ankles, or feet. The stiffness on arising in the morning, which may have been a temporary nuisance, can soon last for hours or even most of the day. You may feel debilitating fatigue that may bother you more than the joint pain. Weight loss is a key symptom of rheumatoid arthritis, even though your eating habits have not changed. Fever, rash, and even internal organ involvement of the heart or lungs can occur with rheumatoid arthritis. These feelings (other than joint pain and the inflammation in other organs) happen when the immune system spills over from the joints to other areas of the body. The exact causes of rashes and heart and lung involvement are not known.

DIAGNOSIS AND TREATMENT

X rays and blood tests can help diagnose rheumatoid arthritis and sort out this cause of pain from fibromyalgia symptoms. Treatment is available, which is more specific than the treatment for fibromyalgia. For instance, anti-inflammatory drugs are helpful to reduce joint inflammation and pain, and many medications are available to control the joint swelling and help prevent long-term damage. If left untreated, rheumatoid arthritis can cause permanent changes in the joints.

Systemic Lupus Erythematosus (SLE or Lupus)

For patients who suffer with fibromyalgia and systemic lupus erythematosus, getting up each morning is a major task. This inflammatory-type arthritis is most common in younger women, ages twenty to forty, and is more common in African-American women. More than 90 percent of systemic lupus erythematosus cases in the United States are women.

WHAT IS SYSTEMIC LUPUS ERYTHEMATOSUS?

In SLE, the body reacts to certain proteins, which it recognizes as foreign. This reaction causes certain cells to create inflammation through cytokines, which are released. The cytokines give "messages" to cause arthritis in the joints. Yet, with SLE, the inflammation is not only in joints, but also commonly in many internal organs, especially the kidneys. There is inflammation in the blood vessels that can cause serious damage to many organs. Fever, rash, heart disease, seizures, blood disorders, and many other complications can happen that could be life threatening.

SIGNS AND SYMPTOMS

The symptoms of SLE are similar to other types of arthritis. You will feel pain in many joints, fatigue, and stiffness in the morning. Rashes are common, including the *"butterfly rash"* across the cheeks in about 15 to 20 percent of cases. There may be an unusual sensitivity to sunlight that causes a rash and other illness. Hair loss, discoloration of the fingers or toes when exposed to cold (Raynaud's phenomenon), and other internal organ damage can occur. Half of those with SLE also have kidney disease. Coexisting blood disorders can cause anemia and blood clots. Chest pain from heart and lung inflammation can happen and seizures or strokes can occur.

DIAGNOSIS AND TREATMENT

Blood tests, especially the antinuclear antibody test (ANA), can help in diagnosing SLE. About 95 percent of active cases of SLE have positive ANA blood tests, although everyone with a positive blood test does not have SLE. ANAs or antinuclear antibodies are found in patients whose immune systems are prone to cause inflammation against their own body tissues. Once your doctor evaluates the clinical findings and blood tests from the examination, she can decide if your symptoms suggest SLE and start you on the proper treatment.

Polymyalgia Rheumatica

Janell, another fibromyalgia patient, had just taken early retirement from teaching when she noticed a sudden onset of severe pain and stiffness in the muscles around her shoulders, upper arms, hips, and thighs. This sixty-two-year-old woman said it was hard to get out of bed because she felt so exhausted and stiff. When she began to run a low-grade fever and experienced weight loss, she called for an appointment.

To make the diagnosis, I used blood tests, such as the blood sedimentation rate, to see if other diseases were present. With polymyalgia rheumatica, the results of this blood test are very high. I also wanted to make sure no other diseases were present, such as temporal arteritis, a disease caused by inflammation in the arteries, that has different treatment.

Once Janell had a proper diagnosis, I treated the arthritis with a COX-2 Super Aspirin (page 78), along with low doses of prednisone to decrease inflammation. I reviewed her fibromyalgia treatment regimen, and she was progressing well using the 7-Step Program. She is now enjoying her active retirement, including travel.

Back Pain

Back pain is the reason Shannon initially came in for an evaluation about ten years ago. At the time, this mother of three could hardly bend over because of sharp, throbbing pain in her back muscles. Even though fibromyalgia was not a common diagnosis in the early nineties, I knew that was Shannon's problem, especially when she described the overall aching, constant fatigue, and feelings of depression.

However, this time Shannon's back pain was different as she described pain and stiffness when she got up in the morning or after she had been sitting at work during the day. After doing some X rays, I found that Shannon had osteoarthritis, a common cause of back pain, which may be sharp or dull and aching. This type of back pain can come on years after an injury as joints that are injured have a higher chance of developing arthritis later. The pain may start slowly then increase over the years as the cartilage of the spine becomes more worn.

WHAT IS BACK PAIN?

I see many fibromyalgia patients of all ages with other causes of back pain, whether from a past injury, poor posture, computer strain, or arthritis. Back pain sufferers have great company as this common health problem affects men and women no matter what their age or occupation, from those who do heavy labor to people who do desk work.

Back pain happens at the most inconvenient times and often for the slightest reasons. For instance, back pain can strike when you bend down to lift a heavy box or even when you simply turn over in bed at night. Some patients tell of getting back pain when they bend over to kiss their children good night or when they lean down to tie their shoes.

Sometimes the pain is called "acute lower back (lumbar) strain," but many times the cause is not apparent at all. At times, there may be pressure on a nerve in the lower back. Specific medical problems, including fracture of one of the bones in the spine due to osteoporosis (thinning of the bones), infections in the spine, internal organ disease, and cancer, can cause acute back pain and are important to find. While this may be the case, sometimes the pain happens when there is no lifting at all—just leaning over. One patient told us that the pain could come on if he leaned over to pick up a feather!

SIGNS AND SYMPTOMS

With back pain, you may notice stiffness when you awaken in the morning or after sitting for more than a few minutes. Other common symptoms include the following:

- Severe pain (sharp, shooting, or the electric-shock type) in the back
- Pain that is felt in the lower back and down the back of one leg
- Pain that worsens with movement or activity
- Numbness or tingling
- Inability to point or extend the big toe on the foot that has leg pain
- Weakness of certain leg or foot muscles
- Disturbance of the normal heel-toe gait, i.e., inability to walk on one foot (or foot-drop)
- Severe pain (sharp, shooting, or the electrical-shock type) in the back of neck, shoulder, or down one arm
- Pain that worsens with movement or activity

- Numbness or tingling in one arm (with neck pain)
- Weakness of arm muscles (with neck pain)

DIAGNOSIS AND TREATMENT

After a thorough physical examination and medical history, your doctor will diagnose the cause of back pain using tests such as X ray, magnetic resonance imaging (MRI), myelogram, or computerized tomography (CT) scan. Depending on the cause, the treatment will be aimed at resolving the specific cause of back pain, along with the fibromyalgia symptoms.

Warning: When to See Your Doctor

See your doctor if . . .

- the back pain is worse with a cough or sneeze
- the back pain or numbness travels down one or both legs
- the pain awakens you from sleep
- you have back pain and it becomes difficult to pass urine or to have a bowel movement
- there is loss of control of the urine or bowel movements

These problems may be the earliest signs of serious nerve damage or other serious medical problems and need early treatment for the best results.

Lumbar Disc Disease

This common problem happens when material in a disc ruptures and presses on a nerve as it travels down the leg. You may feel lower back pain that travels down one or both legs. Diagnosis is made by X ray and other testing such as MRI. Lumbar disc disease is treated with medications, injections, and surgery for relief.

When osteoarthritis or other problems cause narrowing of the spinal canal that contains nerve roots coming from the spinal canal, lower back pain can be severe. This pain may be caused by lumbar stenosis. There is often pain in both legs after walking a short distance with relief of the pain after resting a few minutes. This can be treated with medications, or you may require surgery for relief.

Your Fibromyalgia Action Plan

No matter how much pain you feel with fibromyalgia and other pain-related ailments, you can begin to master this just as you do other areas of your life. In many cases, you can prevent common types of pain. For instance, staying at a normal weight and

	FMS	Osteo-arthritis	Rheumatoid Arthritis	Bursitis/ Tendinitis	Chronic Back Pain	Lumbar Disc Disease
Joint pain	Yes	Yes	Yes	Yes	Yes	Yes
Joint damage	No	Yes	Yes	No		
Inflammation	Uncommon	Yes	Yes	Yes	Less common	Less common
Stiffness	Yes	Yes	Yes	Yes	Yes	Yes
Muscle pain	Yes	Less common	Yes	Yes	Yes	Yes
Fatigue	Yes	Less common	Yes		Yes	
Body aches	Yes	Yes	Yes	Yes	Yes	Yes
Anxiety	Yes	Less common	Yes			
Depression	Yes	Less common	Common	Common	Common	
Interrupted sleep	Yes	Yes	Yes	Yes	Yes	Yes

exercising to keep your back strong will help you prevent many types of back pain. Stopping frequently to stretch and exercise your wrists while using a computer can help you avoid carpal tunnel syndrome. Likewise, avoiding falls and other injuries and exercising may help you avoid problems associated with osteoarthritis.

If you are still suffering with pain even after starting the 7-Step Treatment Program for fibromyalgia, talk to your doctor about other possible causes of pain. Getting an early and accurate diagnosis and the proper treatment can help you to feel pain free so you can begin to enjoy your life again.

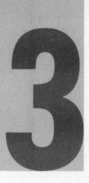

3

MAKING THE DIAGNOSIS

With today's high-tech medicine, we have become used to special testing, blood tests, or other expensive tests to arrive at a diagnosis. However, most laboratory tests are not very helpful by themselves in making the diagnosis of fibromyalgia. In fact, this is one medical problem in which talking with the patient may be the most important tool in arriving at the correct diagnosis. The reason for this is that the major points for diagnosis of fibromyalgia are discovered from the way that you feel. While a physical examination will show your doctor the painful trigger points, as discussed on page 62, even with trigger points you must *tell* your doctor of the exact pain you feel in those areas.

Maria came to see me after living with undiagnosed chronic muscle pain for more than six years. At age thirty-seven, this mother of three told of sleeping all morning after getting her children off to school, taking another late-afternoon nap while her children watched TV, then going to bed before 8:00 P.M. When she wasn't sleeping, Maria described symptoms of chronic headache, irritable bowel syndrome, muscle tension, and tender areas that were painful when anyone touched her.

After ruling out other diseases, Maria was diagnosed with fibromyalgia. Even though she realized that there was no cure for this disease, Maria was relieved to know finally what was causing her daily discomfort and fatigue.

Another patient, Susan, had to face a great deal of anger that it had taken so long to make a diagnosis of her chronic sleep problems, depression, and muscle pain. "If I had known then what I know now, I wouldn't have spent more than two thousand dollars trying to find an answer. Half the battle of winning with this disease is knowing that you didn't make it up."

A Difficult Diagnosis

Many patients like Maria and Susan tell of traveling from doctor to doctor with fibromyalgia—without results—because there are no specific tests for the disease. It may be difficult to make an accurate diagnosis if you cannot see a scientific measurement, such as laboratory tests of X rays. This is why in years past, millions of cases were misdiagnosed as depression or chronic fatigue syndrome (CFS).

Upon evaluation, your doctor will want to have a few basic laboratory tests taken to be sure no other serious medical problems are present. But these tests are limited in number and can be performed at your doctor's office or your local laboratory. They can usually all be done at one visit.

Specific Laboratory Tests Used

Some specific blood tests that your doctor may ask for include a complete blood count (CBC). This test measures hemoglobin levels and provides a count of red blood cells, white blood cells, and platelets. It is used to diagnose many common blood disorders, such as anemia, that can cause fatigue.

The chemistries in your blood will also be checked and will include blood tests that tell how the kidney and liver are functioning, cholesterol and other fats in the blood, calcium levels, and tests of other chemicals such as glucose, that can create problems similar to fibromyalgia, but are treated differently. Thyroid tests will be done at the same time with blood tests to see if the thyroid is working properly. Other laboratory tests may include Lyme disease tests, prolactin level, and calcium level (parathyroid abnormalities).

Testing for Arthritis

If arthritis is a question, one test that may be included is the *erythrocyte sedimentation rate* (sed rate or ESR). This is an old test that measures the rate at which red blood cells settle out in a tube of unclotted blood; a higher than normal sed rate indicates inflammation. Patients with rheumatoid arthritis and other similar types of arthritis have abnormal sed rates. Patients with osteoarthritis and fibromyalgia, however, usually have normal sed rates. Some infections can also cause an abnormal sed rate; the test is not specific for any one disease.

Your doctor may also ask for another blood test to look for *rheumatoid factor.* Rheumatoid factor is an abnormal protein in the blood present in 70 to 80 percent of patients with rheumatoid arthritis. However, rheumatoid factor can also be present in otherwise normal persons.

Your doctor also may test for *antinuclear antibody* (ANA). Like the rheumatoid factor, ANA is an abnormal protein in the blood and is most commonly found with systemic lupus erythematosus. Lupus is a type of arthritis more commonly found in women, especially younger women. It can cause pain and fatigue, and may also cause internal organ problems, such as kidney disease, heart disease, or problems in the brain.

More than 95 percent of patients with lupus have a positive blood test for antinuclear antibody. However, the test can be positive in persons who do not have lupus or who have other, unrelated diseases. The ANA test is important, but there are usually other clues present as well for your doctor.

X Rays Show No Abnormality

X rays of the painful areas will show no abnormality, because the pain caused by fibromyalgia is in the soft tissues (muscles and tendons), which do not show up well on routine X rays. If you have another problem, such as arthritis, then there may be some abnormalities on the X rays to indicate what type of arthritis is present. Keep in mind that fibromyalgia does not cause X ray changes.

Most patients have multiple tests in hopes of finding the answer to their pain. When the pain and fatigue linger with no relief, you may even put added pressure on your doctor to order tests. Sometimes an MRI is used to eliminate other problems, especially if back or neck pain is involved. Yet when these sophisticated and expensive tests are reported with no new answers, your frustration may escalate.

It is important that you talk openly with your doctor in order to interpret the overall results of the total work-up, including the physical examination, laboratory testing, and X rays. This will allow you to have a good understanding of your problems and will provide the basis for your knowledge of the plan of treatment. At this time, be certain to ask any questions and even ask for printed information to read, if you feel the need.

Trust your doctor to decide which set of tests is best in your case to ensure no other medical problems are present. This can help you avoid extra testing that will add little to your diagnosis and only add expense. Also trust your doctor to continue to monitor for other new problems, so you can spend your time more effectively to diminish the pain and fatigue. If there is one specific diagnosis you fear, such as cancer, be sure you tell your doctor. If you still do not feel comfortable with the diagnosis, talk to your doctor and have more testing. Or get a second opinion until you have peace of mind that the problem has been diagnosed correctly. At that time, proper treatment can begin.

Diagnostic Guidelines

Once other medical problems have been ruled out by laboratory tests and X rays, making the diagnosis of fibromyalgia may still be difficult. There are, however, some other guidelines and diagnostic criteria physicians use to determine the problem.

FROM THE AMERICAN COLLEGE OF RHEUMATOLOGY CRITERIA FOR CLASSIFICATION OF FIBROMYALGIA

1. History of widespread pain for at least three months
   Pain in left side of body
   Pain in right side of body
   Pain above waist
   Pain below waist

In addition, pain must be present in one of the following areas:
   neck (cervical spine)
   front of the chest (anterior chest)
   middle of the back (thoracic spine)
   lower back (lumbar spine)

2. Pain in eleven of eighteen tender or trigger point sites on examination

    The locations of the tender point sites are shown in figure 3.1. These are areas of localized tenderness, much more tender than the surrounding areas. They are often present at tendons, in the soft tissues over bones, and in muscles.

Patients have fibromyalgia if criteria from both classification lists 1 and 2 are present. If a patient has another type of arthritis, she may still be classified as having fibromyalgia if she fulfills criteria from both 1 and 2. For example, it is common for a patient with rheumatoid arthritis or systemic lupus erythematosus also to be diagnosed with fibromyalgia due to generalized pain and tenderness. Once fibromyalgia is diagnosed, treatments are available to help the pain, which are separate from treatments for the other chronic diseases.

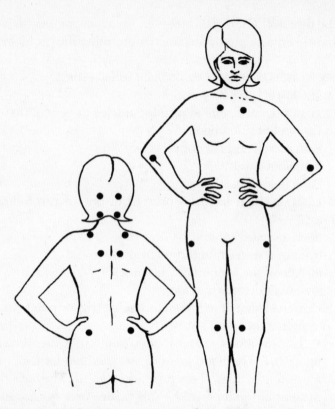

Figure 3.1. Trigger areas are tender points over the neck, shoulder blades, lower back, elbows, and knees or other areas. At least eleven of the eighteen trigger points are found to be painful in patients with fibromyalgia.

Fibromyalgia Evaluations

1. Evaluate widespread pain
2. Evaluate trigger points
3. Ask about fatigue
4. Inquire about sleep disturbances
5. Evaluate stress levels
6. Test for depression

1. EVALUATE WIDESPREAD PAIN

As explained in chapter 1, patients tell of feeling pain "every-where," or at least in so many places that it seems to be every-where. The pain can be sharp, dull, aching, sticking, or pressurelike, or it may be difficult to characterize. The pain often comes from deep within the muscles or joints, as well as from the tendons and ligaments around the joints. Quite often people mistake this pain for a type of true arthritis because of the discomfort and stiffness.

However, the pain from fibromyalgia seems to be from *around* the joints more often than from the joints themselves. Unlike the pain that you may feel after engaging in exercise or a day of housecleaning, which goes away after you walk around, patients tell of pain being present day and night. It makes itself known in the morning on arising and stays all day, even worsening as the day goes on.

Pain is typically felt in the back, neck, arms, and legs, including the shoulders and elbows as well as the hips and buttocks. There may also be pain felt in the hands, wrists, knees, ankles, and feet. Pain in the head and jaw can cause headaches.

Understanding acute and chronic pain. Acute pain is important because it brings to your attention a problem that might cause damage to the body. Acute pain could be a toothache from a cavity, a broken bone, a headache from a sinus infection, or a backache from a strain. Muscle pain, joint pain, and pain in the stomach could all be acute signals of a potential problem. Some injuries can cause acute pain, such as the pain associated with bursitis and tendinitis. Each of these types of acute pain runs its course and disappears as the problem is relieved.

Surveys have shown that more than 70 percent of Americans have acute pain from headache at some time each year, and more than 50 percent have backaches. These pains usually last a few days to weeks. When the problem is relieved, or the injury heals, the pain leaves. For example, acute back pain, the most common cause of loss of work except for the common cold, can come on suddenly and can be severe, but in more than 80 percent of cases it goes away in about two weeks.

Researchers consider acute pain that lasts one to six months longer than expected to be *chronic,* depending on the problem that causes the pain. For example, a back injury causes acute pain; if the pain is no better after three months, it is called chronic back pain. Pain that returns over and over for months or years can be considered chronic. Back pain that is severe and returns many times over one or more years is called chronic back pain. Pain from fibromyalgia is chronic; it lasts for at least three months.

Widespread pain felt all over. Pain is also commonly felt in the abdomen, along with cramps, diarrhea, and constipation. Pain in the bladder area, along with frequent urination, is common. Menstrual periods may be much more painful than usual. Pain may be felt in the chest and may be difficult to tell from pain due to heart disease.

The American College of Rheumatology found that almost all fibromyalgia patients have widespread pain above the waist, below the waist, on the right and left sides of their bodies, and in the neck or back areas. Indeed, people with fibromyalgia may have more pain receptors than others or might be overly sensitive to everything. One patient said just taking a warm bubble bath was a painful experience. The symptom of widespread pain is important in making an accurate diagnosis and in telling the difference between fibromyalgia and other problems.

Temporomandibular joint syndrome. In addition to pain all over, most fibromyalgia patients have jaw pain or pain around the area of the temporomandibular joint (TM). In fact, a majority of fibromyalgia patients have enough pain to be diagnosed with temporomandibular joint (TMJ) syndrome, the most common cause of pain in the jaw and nearby areas of the face and neck. TMJ syndrome and related disorders generally affect younger adults between the ages of twenty and fifty, and, like fibromyalgia, they occur more frequently in women. Some new federal studies estimate that many patients with TMJ spend as much as $500,000 out of pocket seeking relief for this painful syndrome.

With TMJ, pain can be felt in the joint itself just in front of the ear. On the other hand, pain might be felt in the side of the face, head, or neck. You might experience muscle pain or tenderness in the face, ear, neck, or shoulders, and headaches, which are often related to abnormal grinding of the teeth (bruxism). There is usually tenderness in the jaw muscles around the joint, and you may feel a sensation of cracking in the jaw when the mouth is opened. This jaw pain can happen alone from muscle tenderness, or it can be part of fibromyalgia. If conservative treatment, discussed on page 258, does not work to alleviate your TMJ, or if your jaw is locking in place (a sign of disc displacement), call your doctor for further evaluation.

Finding underlying problems. Internal organ problems can cause chronic pain that may mimic the overall aching or throbbing muscle pain of fibromyalgia. If the pain is caused by kidney disease, stomach disease, or other internal organ abnormality, correcting the basic problem will remove the pain. Thus, it is necessary to find and treat any underlying causes of pain before starting treatment for what may seem to be pain from fibromyalgia.

For example, Colleen, a forty-seven-year-old woman, had chronic back pain for more than six months. She had been evaluated for ruptured lumbar disc, but the tests were negative. At that point, she read about fibromyalgia and immediately assumed that this was the proper diagnosis for her pain. However, further testing showed that she actually had a problem with gallbladder disease. After surgery on the gallbladder, her chronic back pain went away completely.

Another middle-aged woman came to our clinic with pain in the lower back and hip area that had lasted for months and had gradually become worse. When it began keeping her awake for several nights in a row, she became worried and sought further help. She was found to have cancer that had spread to the bones of the spine. After starting immediate treatment, she was free of pain.

2. EVALUATE TRIGGER POINTS

In 1990, the American College of Rheumatology established specific diagnostic criteria that require the presence of specific tender or trigger points that are painful to touch when pushed or palpated. In fact, these trigger points are key diagnostic features of the disease (see figure 3.1).

Trigger points, as discussed in chapter 1, are small, localized areas in muscles and tendons that are very tender to pressure in persons with fibromyalgia. These trigger areas are much more sensitive than other nearby areas. In fact, pressure on one of the trigger points with a finger causes pain that makes the person flinch or pull back. The actual size of a trigger point is usually very small, about the size of a dime. Trigger points are scattered over the neck, back, chest, elbows, hips, buttocks, and knees (see figure 3.1), and eleven or more of these are found in most patients with fibromyalgia.

In some conditions other than fibromyalgia, trigger-point pain may be felt in areas away from the actual tender trigger point. For example, pain may seem to travel down one or both legs when trigger areas are pushed in the lower back. This can mimic the pain of pressure on a nerve in the lower back from a ruptured disc, called *sciatica*.

When a physician tests trigger points for pain, he or she will also check *control points* or other nontender points on the body to make sure the person does not react to these as well, which would change the diagnosis. Some physicians use a special instrument, called a *doximeter* or *dolorimeter*, to apply just the right amount of pressure on trigger points.

3. ASK ABOUT FATIGUE

Fatigue has been estimated by researchers to be present at any one time in up to 25 percent of all of us. It can be mild and easily cured by getting extra rest and sleep. But fatigue, tiredness, and exhaustion can be prolonged (lasting more than one month) or chronic (lasting more than six months).

ASSESS YOUR LEVEL OF FATIGUE

Fatigue prevents you from doing normal activities and chores.
You have difficulty making plans due to unpredictable fatigue.
Fatigue is still there after rest or at least eight hours of sleep.
Fatigue interferes with work outside the home.
Fatigue hinders relationship with family members and friends.
You have difficulty getting through the day because of fatigue.
Fatigue prevents exercise or other activity.

This loss of energy is the major complaint of most patients with fibromyalgia and may cause more limitation than the pain. Many patients tell us that if it were not for the fatigue, they could put up with the pain of fibromyalgia.

The fatigue associated with fibromyalgia severely limits daily activities. The tiredness may be especially bothersome in the morning and then improve after a few hours, only to return later in the day. There may be a window of time in each day when activities are tolerated after the morning fatigue wears off but before the afternoon fatigue hits again.

Patients tell of fatigue being most noticeable during activity, which causes immobility as the fatigue becomes more limiting. Fatigue can be even more severe following exercise—it may last days and be so worrisome that a person becomes sedentary.

Fatigue may be worse when a person is physically deconditioned—out of shape. For example, if physical activity has been avoided for a long enough period of time, muscle weakness or tiredness may by itself contribute to fatigue. Researchers have shown that most fibromyalgia patients have below-average fitness levels compared to other persons, and when these people do exercise, they complain of sore muscles without much effort. Many patients with fibromyalgia feel too tired even to work, creating large disability and compensation costs for their employers.

Another condition that can be hard to distinguish from fibromyalgia and causes severe fatigue is *chronic fatigue syndrome* (CFS). In this condition, fatigue lasts more than six months, interfering with daily activities both at home and at work, with no medical problem to explain it.

COMMON SYMPTOMS OF CHRONIC FATIGUE SYNDROME
Relentless fatigue
Memory and concentration problems
Sore throat
Swollen lymph nodes
Muscle and joint pains
Headaches
Poor sleep that is not restful
Exhaustion after exercise

A recent study from the American College of Rheumatology suggests that fibromyalgia and chronic fatigue syndrome may even overlap in the same person. With both conditions, the fatigue and other symptoms seem to increase after periods of high stress or physical exertion. Other studies have indicated that many people who were initially diagnosed as having chronic fatigue syndrome probably have fibromyalgia. After patients started the specific treatment for fibromyalgia, their symptoms lessened dramatically and their energy levels increased.

It may be hard to distinguish between fibromyalgia and chronic fatigue syndrome, as some patients with fibromyalgia tell of symptoms, listed above, that are similar to those of CFS. However, chronic fatigue syndrome patients often have swollen lymph nodes, and the onset of the problem is more sudden. Also, CFS patients don't usually have prominent trigger points of pain.

Your doctor can help you decide what your fatigue indicates, but other medical problems that cause fatigue need to be evaluated and eliminated.

4. INQUIRE ABOUT SLEEP DISTURBANCES

Almost all patients with fibromyalgia complain of sleep disturbances. They tell of waking up frequently during the night and feeling tired and unrefreshed during the day; many require more frequent rest periods during the day. Some researchers find that it may be the constant pain that interrupts sleep.

There is some evidence that sleep disturbances may be caused by an abnormality of deep sleep. Patients tell of feeling awake or in a shallow state of sleep throughout the night, instead of experiencing restful, deep-level sleep. FMS patients also show abnormal brain waveforms in deep sleep. Unfortunately, it is during the delta, or deep-level, sleep that the body does its repair work and replenishment. The hormone *somatostatin,* for example, which is produced in deep sleep and is vital for maintaining good muscle and other soft tissue health, has been found at low levels in fibromyalgia patients. If deep sleep is reduced over a long period of time, the body may have less ability to repair and replenish energy.

ASSESS SLEEP PROBLEMS
Many arousals during a night's sleep
Awakening in the middle of the night
Difficulty in getting to sleep
Reduction in total sleep time
Long awakenings (ten minutes or more) during sleep
Restless legs syndrome during sleep

5. EVALUATE STRESS LEVEL
Evaluating the patient's lifestyle and work habits to see if she is experiencing undue stress or uneasiness each day is an important factor in making a diagnosis. However, which came first: stress or fibromyalgia?

Doctors know that the stress of living with unending, throbbing, or stabbing pain and relentless fatigue can put the patient into overload, resulting in overwhelming feelings of nervousness and anxiety. But they are uncertain as to which came first—a stressful life that brings about the fibromyalgia syndrome or whether having this disease leads to the stress. One study tested fibromyalgia patients on the Hospital Anxiety and Depression Index and a startling 92 percent of patients had a high score. Some consider fibromyalgia to be a psychosomatic illness in which psychological problems, such as depression, disappointment, and anxiety express themselves as physical symptoms, such as backache and sore muscles.

STRESSORS WITH FIBROMYALGIA
Physical stressors (the pain)
Social stressors (loss of friends and activities)
Work stressors (loss of job or difficulty working)
Family stressors (feeling of dependency on others)

No matter which came first, stress can add to problems of anger, distractibility, and irritability and can even lead to further physical changes, such as hypertension or cardiac problems.

ASSESS LEVEL OF STRESS
Various physical symptoms stemming from stress
Feelings of being overwhelmed day after day
Anxiety upon awakening
Impatience for no apparent reason
Inability to sleep soundly
Difficulty in concentrating on projects at home or work
Loss of interest or enjoyment in life
Tendency toward anger or frequent irritability
Changes in appetite (eating more or less food)

6. TEST FOR DEPRESSION
"I don't know if I'm depressed because I ache all over or because I am clinically depressed," Britt said. "I'm not used to being restricted in what I can do and feel caged in by this disease, as if it has a hold on me and won't let me feel free to move like I used to."

Britt told of depression lingering day after day, even when she had everything going for her. She had two healthy children and a husband who was supportive. "Every day I think that maybe this is the day that the sadness will lift. But after tossing and turning each night, I only awaken to more pain and sadness. Will it ever end?"

Again, which came first, fibromyalgia or depression? That question continues to puzzle many researchers, who have found that the two illnesses have similar characteristics. Many people with fibromyalgia are depressed. Conversely, depressed people often complain of inexplainable aches and pains along with fatigue and an inability to stay asleep at night. At some point researchers find depression present in the majority of fibromyalgia patients. In fact, *more than 25 percent* of patients do have depression when fibromyalgia is diagnosed.

When evaluating a patient, the doctor will talk about feelings of depression, as listed below.

COMMON SIGNALS OF DEPRESSION
Disturbances in sleep patterns
Loss of interest in usual activities
Weight loss or gain (more than 5 percent of body weight)
Fatigue
Impaired thinking
Thoughts of dying or suicide
Depressed thoughts or irritability
Mood swings
Staying at home all the time
Avoidance of special friends
Difficulty concentrating
Feelings of worthlessness or excessive or inappropriate guilt
Agitation or, in contrast, a general slowing of intentional bodily activity

Living with the constant pain and fatigue of fibromyalgia can bring about feelings of depression with hopelessness, uncontrollable tearfulness, loss of self-worth, and even suicidal thoughts. Some normal individuals may have one or more symptoms of depression at one time or another. Depression becomes a problem when symptoms begin to occur on a daily basis for a period of at least two weeks and are accompanied by other feelings, such as the fatigue, pain, and muscle aches.

Depression is a very complicated affliction and is not as easy to deal with as other worries and stressors mentioned in this chapter. Often, depression can stem from a biochemical imbalance or can be a symptom of an underlying ailment. Quite often professional help is needed to maintain, control, and cure depression. There are many excellent prescription drugs and many medical protocols that can assist greatly in controlling depression.

Fibromyalgia Can Be Discouraging

These are the most common feelings and signs of fibromyalgia your doctor may consider as he or she makes an accurate diagnosis. I know that these symptoms can be discouraging. The constant muscle pain and fatigue can make daily activities, such as standing, walking, sitting, and even coughing, unbearable. See figure 3.2.

Pain and fatigue lead to inactivity. Because of the disrupted sleep patterns and failure to receive much needed restful sleep, the patient is fatigued even on arising. Daily fatigue can lead to personality changes. A once calm individual will now have a low frustration level, making it difficult to get along at home or work.

With the constant pain and feeling of exhaustion, it is no wonder the patient feels depressed. This in turn can lead to further feelings of discouragement and may create additional social problems and withdrawal from normal activities. Depression may worsen if certain medications, such as tranquilizers to aid with sleep, are used—especially if taken too frequently.

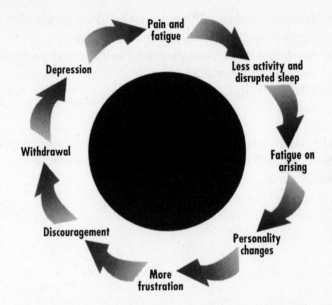

Figure 3.2. Cycle of depression with fibromyalgia

The 7-Step Treatment Program Does Work

The earlier the 7-Step Treatment Program is started, the better the chances are of improvement in a patient's symptoms. The program involves:

1. Experimenting with medications and treatments until a protocol that works is established.
2. Doing specific exercises to reduce muscle pain and increase strength and energy.
3. Learning ways to de-stress and alleviate anxiety at home and in the workplace.
4. Trying a complementary approach to reducing symptoms, including Chinese medicine therapies, homeopathy, chiropractic, acupuncture, massage and therapeutic touch, biofeedback, and herbal therapy, among others.

5. Learning ways to enhance restful sleep and understanding the serotonin/fibromyalgia connection.
6. Starting a nutritional plan for healing using phytochemicals and antioxidants.
7. Understanding the importance of support for symptom relief.

The next seven chapters explain each of these important treatment modalities and, if followed, will enable you to overcome the disabling effects of fibromyalgia.

4

STEP 1:
START WITH MEDICAL TREATMENT

Jacqueline's experience was quite typical of most patients'. She started out with excruciating pain upon arising one morning. She assumed this was a lingering symptom from the flu. Her doctor prescribed an over-the-counter pain medication and told her to drink plenty of fluids and get rest. This thirty-six-year-old interior decorator told of staying in bed for two weeks, putting clients on hold, and farming her children out to friends while trying to get well.

"When I was no better two weeks later," she told me, "I knew I was up against something far worse than the winter flu." Jacqueline went from doctor to doctor, all of whom drew blood for lab work and took many X rays, but to no avail.

"When the last doctor sat me down and went over my chart, he looked at me and said, 'I cannot find anything wrong. You are a well person.' That did it! I knew I was not well, but I was determined to get well."

Jacqueline was diagnosed with fibromyalgia after going over her list of symptoms, including overall deep muscle pain, inability to sleep at night, depression, dizziness, irritable bowel syndrome, urinary frequency, painful menstrual cramps, and headaches. She was put on the 7-Step Treatment Program outlined in this book. While she is not cured—as there is no cure for this disease—she does have more good days than bad days and is able to function and do the things she wants to without debilitating symptoms.

If you have fibromyalgia and live with constant pain and fatigue, like millions of other sufferers, you have probably tried many ways to obtain relief. But to control the pain and other symptoms, you need a multidisciplinary approach. Each step described in the 7-Step Treatment Program is used in conjunction with the others and should be adapted to your lifestyle on a daily basis. Again, the steps will not cure the disease, but they will curb the symptoms.

Start with Moist Heat

Perhaps you have already tried a heating pad at times and found some relief for your aching muscles. I want you to carry this therapy further and use moist heat, twice daily, for ten to twenty minutes on areas of your body that have pain. Twice daily, every day without fail helps relax tense muscles, which makes exercising easier and relieves pain and more.

Because most patients complain of pain all over the body, the most effective and easy-to-use forms of moist heat are a warm shower, hot tub bath, whirlpool, or heated swimming pool. For example, it is easy to put a chair or stool (with rubber tips on the legs for safety) in the shower, then let the warm water permeate the back. Or, if you have access to a whirlpool bath or spa, use it twice daily. Some patients alternate the whirlpool and shower until they find one that is most effective. A warm bath may work for your overall pain, especially the legs and back, but with chronic pain, it may be difficult to sit and then get up from the tub. You don't have to use the same form of heat every time. For instance, you can alternate with a warm shower, whirlpool, bath, or hot towels. Just make sure you stick with the twice-daily plan for optimal pain relief.

If the pain is so intense that you cannot use the shower, whirlpool, or bathtub, then use warm, moist towels or a moist heating pad. Just put the moist towels on the back for a few minutes and change them for warm ones when they cool off. Another choice is hot packs, which can be purchased at a medical supply store. These are heated in hot water, wrapped in a towel, and placed on the back. Some packs are available that can be warmed in a microwave oven. These may be easier to use, but don't allow them to get too hot to touch.

INDIVIDUAL CHOICE OF TREATMENT

You may ignore every treatment suggestion in this book, but DO NOT IGNORE using moist heat, twice daily. The relief from pain that you will feel will make it worth the small amount of time you sacrifice each day.

Choose the form of moist heat that is most convenient and works best for you. Then plan to use it regularly every day. You may quickly find a reduction in pain that will last for a few minutes or hours. Mary Catherine told me emphatically that moist heat did nothing to relieve her pain, but upon questioning, she told me she only used it during her daily shower for ten minutes. Once she began a twice-daily program, she experienced pain relief and was virtually sold on this part of the treatment program.

HELPFUL FORMS OF MOIST HEAT FOR FIBROMYALGIA PAIN
Heated swimming pool
Warm whirlpool or hot tub
Warm shower
Warm tub bath
Hot packs
Warm, moist towel or cloth
Moist heating pad

Add Medications

Certain medications are an effective part of the treatment program for fibromyalgia, along with the twice-daily use of moist heat. Medications can provide much-needed relief of the pain and deep, throbbing muscle aches. In our clinic, we encourage patients to use the lowest dosage possible of any medication and to find the medication that has the fewest side effects. Try to be patient. If pain relief is not experienced with the first medications you try, you and your physician may have to try other combinations. Each of us responds differently to medication, and you'll find that some drugs are more effective than others. There isn't a good way to predict which medication or combination will work best until you try it. Moreover, what works for you might not work for someone else with fibromyalgia.

If you notice unusual symptoms or side effects, stop taking the medication and talk to your doctor.

TRY ANTIDEPRESSANT MEDICATIONS IN FIBROMYALGIA

Many people with fibromyalgia find good relief from a group of prescription drugs that used to be commonly used in high doses to treat depression. These tricyclic and tetracyclic antidepressant drugs are examples of medications that can be used for more than one purpose. The doses used in fibromyalgia are not effective for depression; in fact, they are usually a small fraction of the dose used for depression. However, they are so well known as antidepressants that they are still labeled in that group of treatments. The rationale for their use is twofold—most increase the time spent in stage 4 sleep, and they increase the amount of serotonin in the central nervous system, which has a calming effect. You may want to discuss with your doctor the fact that these are used for depression.

Amitriptyline (Elavil) is one of the most commonly used of these medications. It is one of the oldest antidepressants and has been shown to work well in about one-third of patients. Another bonus is that amitriptyline is very inexpensive. Keep in mind that in fibromyalgia, amitriptyline is used in much lower doses than commonly used for depression. Also, a word of caution: In older people, this medication is usually avoided because of the possible side effects discussed below.

If amitriptyline does not work or has side effects, there are other similar medications to try. Some of the most common are listed on page 76. Be patient during this process of elimination, as it may take two or three weeks before any improvement is shown. You may need to try a number of these medications before you find one that works best for you. However, when you find the right one, you'll know it. There will be a definite reduction of pain, stiffness, and fatigue, and your sleep quality will improve.

Your goal should be to choose the medication that gives the greatest relief with the fewest side effects. About 30 to 60 percent of FMS patients find that one of these medications gives enough improvement that they want to continue taking the drug.

NEWER ANTIDEPRESSANTS MAY HELP

If one of these medications does not give relief of pain and fatigue, there are some newer medications used for treatment of depression that are used in fibromyalgia. These newer medications treat depression by increasing the effect of serotonin, which is thought to be low in fibromyalgia. This group of medicines is commonly called the SSRI (selective serotonin receptor inhibitor) antidepressants. In most cases, newer medications have fewer side effects than the older antidepressant drugs routinely used. Nonetheless, it may take a few weeks to feel an effect on pain and fatigue. And it may still be necessary to try several of the group to see which gives the best effect without side effects.

In some cases your doctor may combine more than one of these medications to try to maximize the positive effect without side effects caused by high doses. Make it your goal to find the right combination that gives improvement in pain and improvement in activity without side effects.

For example, in a study published in the February 2000 issue of the *American Journal of Medicine,* researchers found that FMS patients treated with Prozac (fluoxetine) had improvements in pain, fatigue, and depression compared to those FMS patients in the study who received placebo. Other researchers have combined Prozac with low doses of Elavil (amitryptyline) and found it to be effective in alleviating pain and other symptoms in FMS patients. While other combinations of these antidepressants might help your FMS symptoms, always check with your doctor before you take any of these medications.

Side effects are usually few if lower doses of the medicines are used. The most common side effects are drowsiness (which may help improve the quality of sleep when taken at night), dryness in the mouth, constipation (which is usually not serious), or occasional difficulty in urination. Less common side effects are dizziness, blurred vision, rapid heart rate, or confusion. If you also take other medication, check with your doctor to make sure there are no unwanted problems from the combination of drugs.

SOME OF THE MOST COMMONLY USED ANTIDEPRESSANTS IN FIBROMYALGIA
Ascendin
Celexa
Desyrel
Effexor
Elavil
Norpramin
Pamelor
Paxil
Prozac
Remeron
Serzone
Sinequan
Surmontil
Tofranil
Wellbutrin
Zoloft

TRADITIONAL NONSTEROIDAL ANTI-INFLAMMATORY DRUGS
Often, nonsteroidal anti-inflammatory drugs (NSAIDs) are given to patients with fibromyalgia. Since there is little inflammation with the disease, these drugs usually are not very effective. But these medications can also have some pain-relieving

(*analgesic*) effect that may give relief at times. If you don't find relief from pain after about two weeks, try a different non-steroidal anti-inflammatory drug or acetaminophen (such as Tylenol), which is not a NSAID and is well tolerated by asthmatics and people with gastrointestinal problems.

SOME COMMON TRADITIONAL NONSTEROIDAL ANTI-INFLAMMATORY DRUGS

TRADE NAME	GENERIC NAME
Advil	ibuprofen
Aleve	naproxen
Anaprox	naproxen
Ansaid	flurbiprofen
Arthrotec	diclofenac plus misoprostol
Aspirin products	acetylsalicyclic acid
Clinoril	sulindac
Daypro	oxaprozin
Dolobid	diflunisal
Feldene	piroxicam
Indocin	indomethacin
Lodine	etodolac
Magan	magnesium salicylate
Meclomen	meclofenamate
Monogesic	salsalate
Motrin	ibuprofen
Nalfon	fenoprofen
Naprelan	naproxen sodium
Naprosyn	naproxen
Orudis	ketoprofen
Oruvail	ketoprofen
Relafen	nabumetone
Salflex	salsalate
Tolectin	tolmetin
Trilisate	choline magnesium trisalicylate
Voltaren	diclofenac sodium
Zorprin	zero-order release aspirin (12-hour)

If these drugs give relief, they can be used for a long period of time, but you must always watch for side effects, especially for any upset stomach, since development of peptic ulcers is a possibility. Other serious side effects include dark, sticky bowel movements and blood in the stool. About 1 percent of those who take these NSAIDs for six months or longer have blood in their stool; 2 to 4 percent may develop peptic ulcers and bleeding. To prevent peptic ulcer and bleeding, your doctor may add one of the medicines listed on page 79, the proton pump inhibitors.

THE NEW COX-2 NONSTEROIDAL ANTI-INFLAMMATORY DRUGS (NSAIDs)

If you rely on traditional nonsteroidal anti-inflammatory drugs (NSAIDs)—Advil, aspirin, Motrin, naprosyn—to help ease the deep muscle pain of fibromyalgia, you know how these can often cause stomach distress. NSAIDs work by slowing the action of prostaglandins. These are the chemicals that cause inflammation in arthritis. But prostaglandins also have a positive benefit of protecting the stomach from irritation. Up to now, the available NSAIDs slowed both the bad and good prostaglandins.

The new COX-2 inhibitors or "super aspirins" work in a different way than the older NSAIDs. They stop the "bad" prostaglandins that cause pain and inflammation, while allowing the "good" prostaglandins to do their job protecting your stomach from peptic ulcers. If you take one of the COX-2 NSAIDs, you don't necessarily have to add a proton pump inhibitor.

In our clinic, we find that in addition to the anti-inflammatory effect, the COX-2 drugs can be extremely effective pain medications in most patients. In fibromyalgia there may be little inflammation, so it's no surprise when many NSAIDs don't give much relief. Still, the COX-2 drugs frequently help ease the pain of fibromyalgia, just as they help pain of other related ailments. In fact, COX-2 drugs have been shown to help pain after surgery and tooth extractions and to ease menstrual cramps. Ask your doctor if one of these new COX-2 drugs would help you. In many cases, your doctor may combine these medications with an antidepressant or other medication for maximum effect.

COX-2 NSAIDs
Bextra
Celebrex
Mobic
Vioxx

If you take any of the NSAIDs or COX-2 drugs regularly, you'll need to have a blood test taken every few months to check for side effects. If you have any questions, talk to your doctor before you continue with any NSAIDs.

PRESCRIPTION MEDICATIONS THAT BLOCK ACID PRODUCTION
(PROTON PUMP INHIBITORS)

TRADE NAME	GENERIC NAME
Aciphex	rabeprazole sodium
Nexium	esomeprazole magnesium
Protonix	pantoprazole sodium
Prevacid	lausoprazole
Prilosec	omeprazole

SOME OF THE MOST COMMON SIDE EFFECTS OF NSAIDS
Abdominal pain
Abnormal liver tests (blood tests)
Allergic or unusual reactions
Anemia (lower hemoglobin)
Asthma in those allergic
Blurred vision (occasional)
Bruising and bleeding easily
Confusion
Constipation
Decreased platelet count (can affect bleeding)
Depression
Diarrhea
Difficulty sleeping
Diminished effect of diuretics
Dizziness

Fatigue
Gastritis
Headaches
Heartburn
Hypertension (increased blood pressure)
Impaired thinking (uncommon, but occurs at times in older
    people)
Indigestion
Intestinal bleeding
Itching
Lowered white cells in blood count
Meningitis-like illness (rare)
Mouth ulcers
Palpitations
Peptic ulcers
Rash
Renal (kidney) failure
Sleepiness
Sodium retention with edema (swelling)
Sun sensitivity
Tinnitus (ringing in the ears)

CORTISONE-TYPE DRUGS

Cortisone-type drugs are almost never given regularly by mouth
to fibromyalgia patients, as the side effects of long-term use are
not worth the benefits. On the other hand, local injections of a
cortisone derivative into a painful trigger point can be used.
This type of injection is usually combined with a local anesthetic
and can give good relief from pain at the particular trigger point
that may last from weeks to months (see page 94).

MUSCLE RELAXANTS

Many patients find temporary relief for back and neck pain with
such muscle relaxants as cyclobenzaprine (Flexeril), chlorzoxa-
zone (Parafon Forte), methocarbamol (Robaxin), or cariso-

prodol (Soma). The benefit of muscle relaxants is that they can be used as needed, since they usually give rapid relief that lasts for a few hours. If they don't, then they should be eliminated.

In some clinical tests of FMS patients, Flexeril has been shown to be effective in relieving muscle pain. Although it may work in only 30 to 40 percent of patients, those who find that it helps report getting excellent relief. For those with FMS, Flexeril is often taken at bedtime.

Side effects of muscle relaxants are usually not serious. The most common side effect is drowsiness. It is best to take these only as needed.

MUSCLE RELAXANTS

TRADE NAME	GENERIC NAME
Flexeril	Cyclobenzaprine hydrochloride
Norflex	Orphenadrine
Robaxin	Methocaband
Skelaxin	Metaxalone
Soma	Canisoprodol
Zanaflex	Tizanidine

NONNARCOTIC PAIN MEDICATIONS

Nonnarcotic prescription pain medicines may give relief for hours and can be used when needed. The advantage of this type of medication is that it may not cause the drowsiness or loss of alertness that narcotics can create and is not habit-forming. It is important to be sure that your activity level is improving when you take any type of pain medicines in fibromyalgia. There is no real advantage in simply killing the pain and remaining inactive.

Most who take one of these medications do not have side effects, yet if you try one of them, make sure the medication does not cause nausea. Nonnarcotic pain medications are intended for short-term use (about ten days or less) unless you discuss it with your doctor, so you can monitor for side effects.

Ultracet has been shown in clinical trials to give improvement in pain in fibromyalgia patients. In our clinic, we find that Ultracet (or Ultram), in combination with moist heat, exercises, and other medications, can give wanted relief to many patients. Before you take one of these medications, check with your doctor to be certain there are no interactions with other medications you're taking. In some cases, these should not be combined with antidepressants, especially if you have a history of seizure disorder (epilepsy).

Follow directions on the label, and stop the medication if you have nausea, abdominal pain or upset stomach. If you have a peptic ulcer, ask your doctor before taking these medications.

OVER-THE-COUNTER NONNARCOTIC PAIN MEDICATIONS

TRADE NAME	GENERIC NAME
Advil	ibuprofen
Aleve	naproxen
Many brands of aspirin	acetylsalicyclic acid
Tylenol	acetaminophen

NONNARCOTIC PAIN MEDICATIONS

TRADE NAME	GENERIC NAME
Toradol	ketorolac
Ultracet	tramadol plus acetaminophen
Ultram	tramadol

Follow directions on the label, and stop the medication if you have abdominal pain or upset stomach. If you have had a peptic ulcer, ask your doctor before taking these medications.

NARCOTIC PAIN MEDICATIONS

Narcotic prescription pain medicines are not recommended for routine use in the treatment of fibromyalgia pain. Narcotics can aggravate depression, which can be a part of the fibromyalgia patient's problems.

However, in recent years this group of pain medications has become more accepted for use, particularly when other pain measures don't work. If you follow the program of moist heat, exercises, and the other medications, yet you still don't have relief, talk to your doctor. When carefully given and followed, a narcotic pain reliever can change a life of constant, incapacitating pain and allow you to get around and do the things you want in reasonable comfort. I want you to aim for pain control PLUS improvement in your normal activities and function.

I'll never forget one FMS patient, Linda, a forty-five-year-old mother of four who became severely limited and depressed by the constant pain. Linda became increasingly withdrawn from her family and even shut herself off from her husband of twenty years. After trying about nine different combinations of medications to no avail, Linda finally found excellent control of pain with Oxycontin, a narcotic pain reliever. She now has resumed her full activities with almost no limitations. She knows she must be careful while taking this drug due to its potential for improper use, and she comes to our clinic regularly for evaluation and tests. Linda stays on the 7-Step Treatment Plan, using twice-daily moist heat, exercising regularly, and allowing periodic time-outs throughout her day for de-stressing. The good news is that Linda is now telling her friends that she finally got her life back!

One downside of narcotic pain medications is that they commonly cause constipation. This is easily managed by taking low doses of laxatives and increasing dietary fiber.

MEDICATIONS FOR ANXIETY

Some medicines may help the anxiety brought on by the constant pain and fatigue or by the stress of living with fibromyalgia. Anxiety may accompany depression when it is found along with fibromyalgia, and anxiety may cause worsening of other feelings of fibromyalgia.

Xanax (alprazolam) is used for anxiety and associated depression. In one study, half of the fibromyalgia patients showed improvement with alprazolam and ibuprofen. Although it may take eight to sixteen weeks to feel the full effect of alprazolam, this combination can be tried, especially if anxiety is a major problem with fibromyalgia. Most persons do not have side effects, but watch for sleepiness or decreased alertness.

MEDICINES FOR RESTFUL SLEEP

Prescription sleeping pills can also aggravate depression and often don't give excellent results in most patients. Your doctor can help you decide if they would be helpful in your own situation.

To induce deep sleep states, small doses of one of the antidepressants (see page 76) may be helpful. Sonata or Ambien may also be helpful in fibromyalgia if used under a doctor's supervision.

Help or Hype? New and Experimental Methods of Treating Fibromyalgia

With all the medical research, there are many breakthrough medications and treatments for fibromyalgia—some that are accepted by the medical community and some that draw questions.

As you take new medications or proposed "cures," keep in mind that the power of belief in healing is massive. It was once estimated that about one-third of all healing occurred simply because the patient believed the treatment would work. This is called the *placebo effect*. Some researchers theorize that as much as *two-thirds* of all healing occurs because of the patient's positive beliefs. Placebos have been proven effective in relieving the very real symptoms of colds, headaches, seasickness, angina, anxiety, and postoperative pain.

The following new and experimental treatments may be helpful in your situation. Before you try one, talk with your doctor to see if the treatment is effective. Weigh the effectiveness of the treatment with any side effects. You may want to keep a daily journal of symptoms once you begin the treatment to see if it, in fact, really works.

SAM-e

SAM-e (S-adenosyl methionine), an essential agent in the body, is involved in more than forty biochemical reactions, including detoxification reactions and the manufacturing of antioxidants. Tissue levels of SAM-e decline as we age and in those suffering from depression. Some researchers believe that SAM-e may work as well as prescription antidepressants, as it alters mood and increases restful sleep. While it's not known exactly how SAM-e functions in the body, it's thought that it increases levels of serotonin and dopamine, two brain neurotransmitters.

The beginning study results behind oral SAM-e are quite promising, as this dietary supplement is thought to have anti-inflammatory, pain-relieving, and tissue-healing properties. At least one large study of SAM-e found similar benefit to naproxen, a common nonsteroid anti-inflammatory drug (NSAIDs) prescribed to relieve pain and inflammation. Yet, unlike naproxen or other NSAIDs, SAM-e has fewer side effects. During clinical trials of SAM-e as a treatment for depression, some patients reported marked improvement in arthritis and pain-related diseases.

European doctors have prescribed SAM-e for more than twenty years for depression and pain. If patients cannot tolerate NSAIDs, I sometimes recommend SAM-e to help ease pain and inflammation. Many men and women are able to maintain an active lifestyle using this natural supplement. Nevertheless, SAM-e is quite expensive and may cost you up to $200 per month out of pocket to get relief. As with all dietary supplements, SAM-e should be used cautiously. Follow the package directions, and if you are taking other medication, talk to your doctor before using this supplement.

5-HTP

5-HTP (5-*Hydroxytryptophan*), a derivative of the amino acid tryptophan, is used by the body to increase the central nervous system (CNS) synthesis of serotonin, a powerful neurotransmitter.

Tryptophan is converted into 5-HTP in the body, which then can be converted into serotonin.

As discussed previously, serotonin levels play a significant role in depression, pain sensation, and sleep regulation. For those with fibromyalgia, 5-HTP may help to increase deep sleep and reduce pain. In a study published in *Alternative Medicine Review* (October 1998), researchers reported that supplementation with 5-HTP has been shown to ease symptoms of depression, anxiety, insomnia, and somatic pains in a variety of patients with fibromyalgia. Yet, there are also some small studies showing no benefit at all with 5-HTP. You will have to try it to see if it helps to lessen your pain and other symptoms.

The amount of 5-HTP needed to help reduce symptoms is not known. In some studies, 300 milligrams a day was effective in easing depression. A single 100-milligram dose taken at bedtime seemed to help patients suffering with insomnia. Some studies have shown 400 to 600 milligrams daily of 5-HTP helpful in reducing the frequency of migraine headaches. 5-HTP may interact with some medications, including antidepressants, so as with any dietary supplement, always check with your doctor. As with other over-the-counter natural therapies, 5-HTP is not regulated by the Food and Drug Administration (FDA), so there is no guarantee of the product contents.

MELATONIN

Some patients benefit from the over-the-counter supplement melatonin. In the body, this hormone is produced only at night by the pineal gland in the brain. With sunlight, the body's primary timekeeper, this natural hormone helps to set the brain's biological clock. This clock determines all of the body's circadian rhythms, from hormone releases and body temperature to the sleep-wake cycle and digestive functions.

As a natural supplement, melatonin is available over the counter in drugstore or health food stores. It has been cited in the media as a breakthrough for everything from anti-aging and cancer prevention to treatment of sleep disorders. Even though this hormone is *not* regulated by the FDA, it has been recommended by many researchers as a way to counter the effects of jet lag. The National Institutes of Health is sponsoring $50 million of research on melatonin at this time, yet many of these claims will take years to sort out with scientific studies.

In some sleep research studies, scientists report that melatonin taken an hour before bedtime has been shown to induce sleep more quickly and continue longer than with a placebo. Though melatonin appears to be nontoxic, taking too much or at the wrong time could make you sleepy when you need to be awake! For those with fibromyalgia and the relentless fatigue, being sleepy during the daytime is not a desirable side effect.

At this writing, there is very little evidence as to the long-term effects of melatonin or even the doses recommended. If you want to try melatonin, first talk with your doctor. Then, with your doctor's consent, try a low dose (1 mg) until you get an idea of how you might react. Some patients have reported negative side effects such as grogginess upon awakening, daytime drowsiness, depression, and vivid nightmares.

If you do take melatonin, keep in mind that researchers are still concerned about the unknown side effects associated with natural supplements, as well as the possibility of undiscovered health risks. Actually, some newer studies have found that sweat and heat work much better than any sleep aid. Exercise raises the body temperature when performed in the afternoon, and this extra heat allows the body to go into deeper sleep at nighttime. You can get the same effect with "passive heating," or taking a warm bath several hours before you go to sleep at night.

GUAIFENESIN

For the past several years, guaifenesin, a new "cure" for fibromyalgia, has been touted by some physicians. Although there are no published clinical trials or studies in medical journals showing results of a cure, many patients with FMS claim to have found relief taking this medication. Nonetheless, before you run to the corner drugstore and try to find guaifenesin, it's important to know what it is and what it is intended to do in FMS.

Guaifenesin is not a recent medical discovery. Rather, it is an inexpensive expectorant found in many cough remedies. (Robitussin is an over-the-counter cough medication; Humibid is a prescription product.) Guaifenesin has no significant side effects, and for people with bronchial or lung problems it helps to thin mucus, making it easier to expel.

Proponents postulate that in people with FMS, there is an excess accumulation of phosphates. Guaifenesin helps the kidneys excrete and lower the phosphate levels in the blood. According to those who have tried this medication at the lowest recommended dosage (300 mg, twice a day), symptoms of fibromyalgia intensify during the first few months of treatment, which is said to be a sign of "disease reversal," and then symptoms may subside.

The effects of guaifenesin are said to be blocked by sources of salicylates, including aspirin. If you choose to try this treatment, first talk with your doctor. You may want to follow a strict dietary plan that excludes salicylates from your meals and medications (aspirin), as well as avoid cosmetics and personal hygiene products containing this substance.

Many leading researchers believe that because millions of FMS patients have been told the problems are "mental" in nature, having the hope of a "cure" can give something positive to cling to. Feeling in control of one's health is crucial for wellness, and guaifenesin has given some this type of self-efficacy.

The bottom line is guaifenesin will *not* hurt you and it may help. However, so far, the scientific proof that this medication will cure fibromyalgia is simply not there. Continue to follow your doctor's instructions, report to your regular visits, and ask questions about any highly promoted "cure" for FMS before you opt to use it. On the other hand, if you do find relief with guaifenesin or other nontraditional treatment with no unwanted side effects, more power to you!

NADH

NADH is a naturally occurring enzyme found in all living cells. This enzyme plays a central role in the body's energy-producing capacity. In the past few years, researchers at Georgetown University have treated patients with chronic fatigue syndrome with NADH with promising results. In these clinical trials, patients reported relief from fatigue, along with increased strength and endurance, and a boost in mental and physical energy.

While the jury is still out on the optimal effectiveness of NADH in symptoms of fatigue and muscle aches, the data on this experimental drug look promising.

DETROL AND DITROBAN

As discussed, treating symptoms is the best way to control FMS. Overactive bladder, including symptoms of urinary frequency, urgency, or urge incontinence, is a major concern of many. (Urgency is the sudden, overwhelming urge to urinate; frequency means urinating more than eight times in twenty-four hours; and urge incontinence is the sudden and total involuntary loss of urine.)

Many FMS patients tell of having to change their lifestyle to cope with an overactive bladder to the extent of even reducing fluids or staying inside all day and night. In some cases, having an overactive bladder can result in emotional distress and contribute to depression. Detrol (tolterodine tartrate) is FDA approved for the treatment of overactive bladder.

With Detrol or Ditroban, patients may experience a significant reduction in frequency of urination. The side effects are minimal but may include dry mouth, headache, constipation, indigestion, and dry eyes.

Ask your doctor if one of these medications may help you return to a normal, active life.

MALIC ACID AND SUPER MALIC

In recent years, evidence has been gathered that suggests FMS is the result of local hypoxia to the muscles, meaning patients have low muscle-tissue oxygen pressure in affected muscles. Malic acid, derived from such foods as apples, apricots (both fresh and dried), cherries, plums, and dried dates and figs, may play a key role in energy production, specifically during hypoxic conditions. In some test studies, volunteers with FMS took 1,200 to 2,400 milligrams of malic acid. Within forty-eight hours of supplementation, they had improvement in pain relief. Likewise, upon discontinuation of malic acid for forty-eight hours, the improvement was lost.

Super Malic, a tablet containing malic acid (200 mg) and magnesium (50 mg), is being studied for treatment of fibromyalgia. In scientific studies, volunteers with FMS took a fixed dose of Super Malic. Although no symptom change was seen in short-term trials, when the dose was increased (up to six tablets of Super Malic, twice a day) and continued for a longer duration of treatment in the open label trial, some reductions in the severity of pain and tenderness were found.

Researchers believe that Super Malic is safe and may be helpful in treating FMS. If you try Super Malic with your doctor's consent, consider staying on this therapy for at least two months to receive full benefit.

MAGNET THERAPY

Many with FMS are turning to magnet therapy in an attempt to find treatment for pain without drugs. This form of drugless therapy is used by many athletes and touted for relieving pain within minutes in some cases.

Magnet therapy goes back for centuries. Some believers feel that the magnet stimulates or interacts with the body's electrical system to increase circulation, reduce inflammation, and decrease pain. Others, who faithfully strap magnets onto sore muscles, claim that the magnetic field interferes with the body's pain perception and the magnets stimulate endorphins in the body (natural painkillers).

Quite honestly, no one really knows how magnets work. A surprising study from Baylor College of Medicine revealed that magnets may reduce muscular pain in post-polio patients. Volunteers in the Baylor study said they got pain relief from very low energy magnets (300 to 500 gauss or a little larger than a refrigerator magnet)—once a day for only forty-five minutes.

It would take subsequent studies to make any guarantees, yet even some researchers are strapping magnets to arthritic knees in hopes this experimental treatment works. At this time, the National Institutes of Health has created an office of alternative medicine, which is paying for the magnet studies on fibromyalgia patients.

The downside of magnet therapy is the unknown. The FDA warns doctors about the unknown side effects of magnet therapy. Just as they do not know if magnets can end pain, they don't know if they are harmful either. Some have reported such side effects as headaches, insomnia, and backache after extensive magnet therapy.

It's important to realize that although there is hope for magnet therapy in stopping chronic pain, it is still highly experimental.

HUMAN GROWTH HORMONE

Some researchers suspect that human growth hormone, a hormone secreted by the pituitary gland in the brain, may be related to fibromyalgia. Studies show lower levels of human growth hormone in patients with FMS, even compared to those who suffered from pain but not fibromyalgia.

In one particular study, published in the journal *Arthritis and Rheumatism* (May 2002), researchers at the Oregon Health Sciences University in Portland put twenty women with fibromyalgia and ten normal women through physical stress. The women had to run on a treadmill until exhaustion. Afterward, the normal women had increased levels of human growth hormone, while the women with fibromyalgia did not.

Theorizing that the human growth hormone was blocked by somatostatin, another hormone, the women with fibromyalgia were given a drug, Mestinon, which is normally used for people with certain muscle disorders. After running on the treadmill again, their growth hormone levels increased just like those of the normal women. While Mestinon is not used for fibromyalgia patients, this study does indicate a possible growth-hormone defect with FMS.

Human growth hormone is expensive, available by prescription only, and, in cases of genuine deficiency, has been shown to give important health benefits when taken under a doctor's supervision. However, unsupervised use of any hormone supplement can lead to health problems.

Keep in mind that although these findings may give new insight into the treatment of fibromyalgia, much research remains to be done. Although scientists are hopeful about this connection, it will be some time before new treatments will result.

Other Medical Modalities for Treating Pain

CREAMS, LINIMENTS, AND LOTIONS

Creams, liniments, and lotions are widely advertised and used for the pain of arthritis and other conditions. Many types are available at your drugstore and at health food stores. They are not harmful when used properly and can be continued if you feel improvement in muscle pain.

ARNICA

An herbal ointment available at natural food stores that helps to reduce inflammation and decrease pain. (This natural product may cause skin rash in some allergic people, so use with caution.)

CAPSAICIN

Capsaicin, sold over the counter under various brand names, such as Zostrix, has been found to be quite beneficial in the few existing studies. One form of capsaicin is available in a roll-on applicator and is sold as Capsin (ask your pharmacist for information on this product).

Capsaicin has an active ingredient derived from red chili peppers. When nerve endings in the body are touched by capsaicin, they produce substance P, a neurotransmitter that carries pain messages to the brain. Repeated applications of capsaicin results in fewer pain messages to the brain. While this cream can cause warmth or a burning sensation, it does not cause blistering, and the burning feeling usually decreases the longer the cream is used. Use caution when applying capsaicin as it can burn your eyes, mouth, or nose if you don't wash your hands well. Also, avoid hot baths or showers after applying capsaicin as it may irritate and burn the skin.

BOSWELLIN CREAM

Another popular cream, Boswellin Cream, can be found at some health food stores and has been used for centuries to treat pain-related ailments. This cream is made of four triterpene acids from the herb *Boswellia serrata*, which has been found to bring temporary relief to minor aches and pains associated with arthritis.

Use this cream with caution as it does produce mild inflammation and redness to the skin when applied, supposedly in order to achieve its healing properties. A loose bandage is then used with the cream. Be sure to use this for external use only, and if the skin becomes inflamed, stop its usage.

COMPOUNDED CREAMS

Your pharmacist can compound a special prescription cream, according to your doctor's instructions. This topical salve or gel is applied directly to the site of pain, and helps to alleviate muscle pain for many patients. For the main ingredient, the cream may have ibuprofen, a COX-2 inhibitor, Lidocaine, or even a narcotic pain reliever. The benefit is that the medication goes directly into the site of pain without giving you the side effects of an oral medication.

DMSO

DMSO (Dimethyl Sulfoxide) has been used to treat illnesses in horses for years. In humans, DMSO has been used for injuries to muscles and tendons in athletes. In these athletic injuries, it is applied to the skin, not taken internally.

DMSO is sold in an impure form in some hardware stores. When it is applied to the skin, it is absorbed into the blood, and causes a strong garlic-breath odor. Sometimes the skin is irritated where it is applied. The more dangerous form of DMSO is when it is injected into a vein as it can cause liver or other internal organ damage. This should never be done.

While the FDA has not approved DMSO for use in arthritis or bursitis, it has found that it might be helpful in relieving pain caused by bursitis, acute injuries, and possibly rheumatoid arthritis. Even though not approved by the FDA, DMSO is used by some patients. In my clinic, I see little use among fibromyalgia patients, but I do not object if it is used carefully and gives relief.

LOCAL INJECTIONS

A local anesthetic combined with a low dose of a cortisone derivative can give temporary relief when there are painful trigger points. Within a few days, there is often relief of pain from the localized trigger point and surrounding areas, with relief often lasting weeks at a time. This treatment is especially good when there are one or two trigger points causing major pain and limited movement. Also, if there is improvement in many areas but one or two painful areas remain, then local injection can be very helpful.

There are usually no serious side effects, and there should be no significant problems from an occasional local injection of these areas of tissue pain. This cortisone dose should have little effect on the rest of the patient's body.

OTHER INJECTIONS FOR PAIN

There are several types of injections available other than those used on trigger points. Injections around the spine in specific areas (epidural injections, facet joint injections, and nerve block) using a local anesthetic and a cortisone derivative may give pain relief that lasts for weeks or months. If this has positive results, the injections may be repeated after several months. Sometimes, stopping the pain temporarily may have a lasting effect on the chronic pain.

ULTRASOUND

Ultrasound uses sound waves that are applied to the muscles, tendons, and other soft tissues of the back. This may help relaxation, decrease inflammation, and improve pain in tender points. It is more commonly used for acute back pain and other similar situations than for chronic pain. It can be done properly by your physical therapist and continued if it gives relief.

TENS

Transcutaneous Electrical Nerve Stimulation (TENS) uses electrical stimulation for pain relief from many different causes. Electrical impulses sent to certain nerves block the messages of pain being sent by other nerves from the painful area. These impulses might also cause the body to release *endorphins*, which are natural pain relievers produced by the body.

The person wears a unit, a stimulator and battery, usually on a belt. Electrical wires from the stimulator attach to electrodes held by adhesive, usually a patch, on the skin. The electrodes are placed in the area of pain but may need to be tried at different locations to get the best relief.

The TENS unit can be used continuously or only as needed for the pain. Usually there will be a trial of about one month to see the effect on pain.

LONG-TERM NARCOTIC INJECTION

In unusual cases of some chronic pain, surgery can be used to insert a catheter for long-term use of drugs, such as narcotics, for pain control. A device called a *port* is installed, usually on the abdomen, which allows injections of medication as often as needed. A pump can also be installed through surgery to allow medication (such as morphine) to be delivered continuously for long-term pain relief.

COMPREHENSIVE PAIN CLINIC

As discussed in chapter 10, a comprehensive pain clinic may be useful, but only after you have tried the 7-Step Treatment Program and are still living with pain each day.

Read the criteria for finding a qualified pain clinic on pages 248 to 251, and with your doctor's consultation, choose one that best suits your particular needs.

Combining Other Treatment with Medications

In our clinic, we find that a combination of heat and exercise, along with one of the antidepressant medications and the most effective nonsteroidal anti-inflammatory drug, gives the best relief in the deep muscle pain. I will tell you up front that choosing the medications does require some trial and error. However, it is important that you patiently try the available medications in each group to be sure you have the best chance for success in pain control and increased activity.

Minimize Food and Drug Interactions

There are preventive measures you can take to ensure the least possible interaction between food and the drugs you take. Some medications must be taken immediately following a meal; others must be taken on an empty stomach. Some medications cannot be mixed with alcohol or the end result can be deadly. If you drink alcohol with an antidepressant, for example, the results can be excessive intoxication. Alcohol taken with a muscle relaxant depresses brain activity, and alcohol with a hypnotic/sedative (sleeping pill) causes oversedation and can even be fatal. Carefully follow your pharmacist's instructions on each prescription and over-the-counter medication you take, and be sure to contact your physician if you have any questions concerning medication and possible reactions.

Common Food and Drug Interactions

	Take on empty stomach	Take with food	Avoid alcohol	May increase appetite for carbs	Watch for stomach upset	Causes dry mouth
Acetaminophen (Tylenol)	○		○			
Aspirin (Many brands)		○	○		○	
Amitriptyline (Elavil)		○	○	○		○
Ibuprofen (Advil, Motrin)		○	○	○		
Naproxen (Aleve)		○	○	○		

Trial and Error to Wellness

In short, there is hope to treat fibromyalgia's symptoms. Although there is no quick fix, you can find success with treatment using a trial-and-error procedure. That is, you must work with your physician and try various medications and medical or complementary treatments to find the ones that will help. This will take some time as you sort through the options, but you will see greater benefits in the long run with symptom control, including pain management and less fatigue.

5

STEP 2: EXERCISE DAILY FOR MOBILITY AND ENERGY

Janet spoke of living with the symptoms of fibromyalgia for five years, traveling from doctor to doctor, complaining of widespread pain, tenderness at specific tender points, muscular weakness, and an overall flulike exhaustion. "I think most of them thought that I was this stereotypical hysterical female, but I knew differently. I knew that something was terribly wrong with me," she said.

This thirty-four-year-old mother and homemaker was an avid runner before she had children. "In college I used to run several miles each day before classes," she continued. "Then I started my career and family, and I never found time to exercise. Now I couldn't exercise if I wanted to."

This young woman is characteristic of so many patients, that is, most are aerobically unfit and not engaging in any regular exercise. Research has found that fibromyalgia patients are more than *75 to 80 percent below average in fitness* compared with age- and gender-matched subjects of the general population.

I have heard myriad reasons from patients as to why they avoid exercise, including:

"How can I exercise? I can hardly walk to my car each morning."
"Sure I'd exercise if only I had some energy."

"Exercise frightens me. What if it makes this disease worse?"

"I tried to walk around the block the other day, and it left me exhausted."

"There's no way this tired body can exercise. I can hardly make dinner."

"If I could ever sleep all night without tossing and turning, then maybe I'd feel like exercising."

"If you could cure me of fibromyalgia, I'd be glad to start exercising."

Exercise Is Essential for Muscle Strength and Flexibility

Both as a doctor and as someone who exercises daily, I know that a regular exercise program is essential to keep muscles strong and flexible, to control weight, and to stay active in other areas of life. Aerobic exercise particularly has also been shown to improve symptoms and restore muscle strength in patients with fibromyalgia. In fact, exercise and activity allow patients to have some control over the disease and the amount of pain they feel.

If you want to reduce your pain and get more energy, you'll have to start exercising. More and more studies are confirming the benefit of exercise on fibromyalgia. In one three-year study in Finland published in the journal *Arthritis Care and Research* (August 2001), researchers found that exercise is more effective in easing the symptoms of fibromyalgia than medication or alternative treatments. Investigators reported overall pain and count of the body's tender points declined significantly from the beginning of the study with the biggest changes happening after one year of exercise. Patients also reduced intake of medications, including nonsteroidal anti-inflammatory drugs and antidepressants.

In another enlightening study reported in *Arthritis Care and Research* (April 2002), researchers found that a combination of strength training and aerobic exercise improved women's muscle strength and overall endurance. In the twenty-week study, the women underwent a progressive exercise regimen, starting with pool exercises to improve joint movement. They also walked and did resistance exercises with hand weights, machines, and their body's own resistance. At the end of the program, fibromyalgia patients reported that their overall strength and endurance levels improved, as did their moods, outlook, and pain.

Still, even with the positive reports of exercising halting FMS symptoms, Lou was the most resistant patient I'd ever treated when it came to moving around more. Even though she had successfully followed the other steps in the 7-Step Treatment Program, she simply refused to exercise.

"When I think of moving my legs and arms, all that comes to mind is pain, pain, and more pain," Lou said strongly. "And I'm sick and tired of living with pain."

It took three months to convince Lou that even though the pain wouldn't go away immediately, she would begin to notice a difference in her pain threshold within several weeks of starting her exercise program. And at her six-month visit, Lou found that exercise was the missing link in her treatment. Six months before, this fifty-two-year-old woman could hardly climb up onto the examining table. Now Lou was lifting her arms and stretching down to the floor—without pain.

In our clinic, we see patients who are able to see and feel great improvement with managing symptoms by maintaining a regular exercise program. Not only does exercise slow down the heart-racing adrenaline associated with stress, but those with fibromyalgia experience the added benefit of boosting levels of endorphins (proteins that reduce feelings of pain and induce euphoria), helping to relieve low-grade depression, and also helping them to receive restful sleep.

Exercise Boosts Serotonin Levels

Serotonin is a neurotransmitter in the brain that scientists have found to be related to fibromyalgia. (Neurotransmitters are chemicals that send specific messages from one brain cell to another.) While only a small percentage of all serotonin (1 to 2 percent) is located in the brain, this neurotransmitter is believed to play a vital role in mediating moods.

Studies have found that too much stress can lead to permanently low levels of serotonin, which can create aggression. When serotonin levels are increased in the brain, it is associated with a calming, anxiety-reducing effect, and, in some cases, with drowsiness. Also, a stable serotonin level in the brain is associated with a positive mood state or feeling good over a period of time. Lack of exercise and inactivity can aggravate low serotonin levels.

It also appears that women may have a greater sensitivity to the changes in this brain chemical. Mood swings during the menstrual cycle, menopause, or following the birth of a child may be induced by the action of hormones on neurotransmitters.

Various factors can have a positive effect on serotonin levels, including sunlight, certain carbohydrate foods, some hormones, and exercise. Not only does exercise act as nature's tranquilizer, helping to boost serotonin levels in the brain, but studies have shown that exercise also triggers the release of epinephrine and norepinephrine, which are known to boost alertness. For those who feel stressed-out frequently, exercise will help to desensitize your body to stress.

Before starting an exercise program, most patients experience a cycle of inactivity that usually begins with muscle pain and leads to inactivity, poor physical conditioning, and disrupted stage 4 (delta) sleep. This vicious cycle can be halted with increased exercise and fitness.

Exercise Boosts Serotonin Levels

A revealing study published in the journal *Arthritis Care and Research* (January 2002) concluded that not only does exercise improve the mood of patients with fibromyalgia, it also helps to increase physical function. In the study, exercisers reported less depression at six, twelve, and twenty-three weeks while depression scores in the comparison group (nonexercisers) stayed unchanged. The exercisers received another bonus—they were

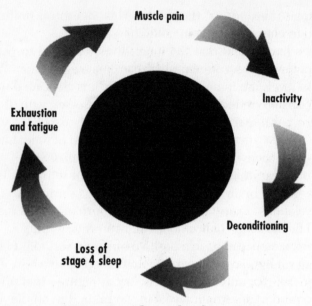

Figure 5.1. The cycle of inactivity

able to increase the distance they could walk by almost one-half mile more per hour than previously. Again, the nonexercisers did not have this benefit.

Exercise Helps You to Maintain a Normal Weight

Being overweight is a hindrance for those with fibromyalgia. Additional weight can keep you from being active, hinder your sleep, and make you feel more depressed. Your weight can depend on many variables, including height, age, bone structure, and weight-cycling history. In the past, height/weight charts gave an accurate portrayal of overweight. However, experts now believe that your body mass index (BMI) may give a more accurate picture of health. BMI is your body weight (in kilograms) divided by your height (in meters squared). The BMI number or value correlates to your risk of adverse effects on health, with higher numbers showing an increased risk.

According to the American Dietetic Association, people with a higher percentage of body fat tend to have a higher BMI than those who have a greater percentage of muscle.

Here's how to figure out your BMI:

1. Write down your weight in pounds _____.
2. Multiply that number by 703: ____ × 703 = _____.
3. Multiply your height in inches by itself: ___ × ___ = ____.
4. Divide the answer to number 2 by the answer to number 3 to get your BMI _____.

Comprehensive research reveals that maintaining a normal body weight is important for staying well and avoiding chronic illness such as diabetes or heart disease. Staying at a normal weight may also play a role in the pain you feel. In a study published in the *Scandinavian Journal of Rheumatology* (March 2002), investigators concluded that weight loss might improve physical functioning in those with fibromyalgia. In the study, researchers compared FMS symptoms at different levels of BMI and found that the higher the BMI, the greater the symptoms of fatigue and painful trigger points.

As you seek to maintain a normal weight, it's important to understand that each person is different. While your best friend may be the same height as you, yet weigh ten to twenty pounds less, you both may be at your optimal weight, depending on certain variables, including height, age, bone structure, and genetics.

Exercise is a proven way to burn calories, build muscle, and reduce excess weight. Keep this in mind the next time you put on your walking shoes. Not only will you look and feel better, you will have fewer pain symptoms and less fatigue after exercise.

BMI CATEGORIES

20–25	normal weight
26–29	overweight
30 and above	obese

Exercise: Safe and Necessary

Until recently, many researchers felt that exercise might exacerbate fibromyalgia's symptoms or accelerate the disease; thus, physicians encouraged patients to seek rest, not activity. But more recent scientific tests are conclusive in determining that, for most patients, range of motion, strengthening, and aerobic conditioning exercises are safe and necessary.

Most patients have a reduced quality of life, which can be the result of impaired endurance. Because of this, exercise is one of the first modes of treatment I encourage patients to undertake in order to reduce pain, improve endurance for physical activities, improve cardiovascular fitness, and cope with life's stressors, including their disease, in a more accepting manner. In fact, I have found that most patients can push themselves to exercise, even if they have not exercised for years and are in some pain.

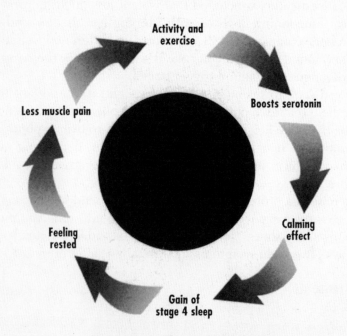

Activity and exercise

Boosts serotonin

Less muscle pain

Calming effect

Feeling rested

Gain of stage 4 sleep

Figure 5.2. The cycle of activity

If you are considering undertaking the recommended exercise program described in this book, I urge you to consult first with your physician to determine that it is safe to exercise.

BENEFITS OF REGULAR EXERCISE FOR FIBROMYALGIA PATIENTS
- Improves sense of well-being
- Strengthens bones
- Strengthens muscles
- Gives range of motion to painful muscles and joints
- Increases aerobic capacity
- Improves quality of sleep
- Stimulates growth hormone secretion
- Burns calories and makes weight control easier
- Increases cardiovascular health
- Reduces anxiety levels and depression
- Secretes endorphins or "happy hormones"
- Improves outlook on life
- Relieves stress associated with a chronic disease
- Increases energy
- Places the responsibility of healing in the hands of the patient

Different Types of Exercise

As you begin your exercise program, you will focus on three different types of exercise:

Range-of-motion or stretching exercises. These involve moving a joint as far as it will go (without pain) or through its full range of motion. The range-of-motion exercises or stretching will help you maintain flexibility in your muscle groups.

Endurance or conditioning exercises. When you increase your endurance threshold with cardiovascular forms of exercise, such as walking, biking, or swimming, you will not only strengthen your muscles, but also condition your body and build coordination and endurance.

Strengthening exercises. These exercises help to build strong muscles and tendons needed to support your joints. I recommend cautiously performing strength training using either resistance machines, resistance bands, or free weights (handheld weights that are not part of a machine).

Range-of-Motion or Stretching Exercises

Flexibility, the ability to move your joints through their full range of motion, is one of the key elements of fitness, along with cardiovascular endurance and muscle strength. Yet most patients have become inflexible because they have avoided exercise due to fatigue. This condition varies from one person to the next, as one patient may be flexible in her spine yet stiff in her shoulders. Another person may be able to bend down and touch the floor yet not be able to bend from side to side without pain and stiffness. Being flexible also helps protect you from joint injury, and the best way to get this protection is through stretching before activity or exercise.

More than anyone, sedentary people need the relief from muscle tension and stiffness that stretching provides. When done correctly, stretching feels good and is healing. Not only does a stretched muscle experience an increase in muscle tone, mobility, and greater circulation along with a marked decrease in pain, but also is less likely to be injured. Improper or excessive stretching, however, may actually increase the likelihood of injury—something you want to avoid with a chronic pain disease.

SEEK INSTRUCTION FROM A PHYSICAL THERAPIST

Because fibromyalgia's symptoms are physiologic in nature, you may want to seek instruction from a licensed physical therapist. These professionals have a background in anatomy and *kinesiology* (study of movement), allowing them to develop specific stretching and strengthening programs for your specific needs.

Physical therapy can enable you to regain control of your illness as you focus on lifestyle changes rather than on the chronic dysfunction. Proper posture, which your physical therapist will help you with, allows efficient muscle function, thus avoiding undue fatigue and pain. The slow stretching exercises below, performed *after* the application of moist heat, will improve muscle flexibility and reduce muscle tension.

Be sure that symptom relief modalities, such as heat and gentle massage, are only used for brief periods of time and in preparation for active exercise.

STRETCH MORE, HURT LESS

What's the first thing you do when your stomach growls? If you're like me, you grab a snack or refreshing drink to calm the hunger pangs. Well, what do you do when your body feels sluggish, achy, or stiff? If you're like many fibromyalgia patients with chronic pain, you rest. That is not the appropriate response! To offset the muscle pain and stiffness, I want you to get up and start stretching those tight muscles. Stretching not only improves circulation to the muscles and joints, but also increases your range of motion so that moving around becomes easier in time.

While there is some debate in the medical community about the need to stretch before exercise, some new findings reinforce the belief that preworkout stretching can help to prevent injury. In a study to find out if stretching caused inflammation in the muscle, researchers found the opposite: passive stretching protects the muscle from injury. In the study presented at the Experimental Biology 2002 conference investigators reported that injury-preventing immune system inflammatory cells called *neutrophils* were seen in large numbers among the passive-stretching muscle fibers. It is thought that these neutrophils have a protective effect on the muscle, helping to block injury during exercise.

Your stretching routine should be specific and include all the major muscle groups, including shoulders, hips, pelvis, buttocks, thighs, and calves.

Begin your stretching regime with five minutes of walking in place until your body warms up. This enables sore, tight muscles to loosen up. Then work at stretching one muscle at a time, holding your stretch for at least thirty to sixty seconds. A word of caution: Avoid overdoing this, as you don't want to add more damage to your aching muscles.

Although it is important to get to the point where you can do stretches daily, you must make a conscious effort to do the exercise correctly in order to obtain optimal benefit. It is better to do only a few stretches correctly than to hurry through them and risk injury.

Again, if stretching is done right, it should feel good. If you experience pain, check with your physician or physical therapist. The goal of stretching is to *decrease* pain and immobility, not increase it.

For more information about how to stretch properly, check with a physical therapist in your area. You can seek recommendations from your physician or contact the Private Practice Section, American Physical Therapy Association (see Resources, page 286).

The following exercises are designed to build flexibility and strength in the neck, shoulders, arms, back, and elbows. It is important to work toward a goal of doing these exercises twice a day, twenty repetitions each. At first you may only be able to do one to two repetitions of each exercise. That's a reasonable start. But as you gain strength and mobility, move into a twice-daily, twenty-repetitions-each routine. If you have any pain or unusual feeling, stop the exercise and contact your physician.

Sometimes it is helpful to have some gentle assistance from a family member or friend. Your physician or physical therapist can show you how.

A word of caution: Do not hold your breath while performing any exercise. If you feel pain with any of the suggested exercises, stop the exercise and discuss it with your physician.

Neck Range-of-Motion Exercises

It is important to build strength in the neck as well as improve its mobility and flexibility. Because fibromyalgia causes stiffness and pain, these range-of-motion exercises will enable your body to perform more effectively. Although flexion should be done while standing, the rest of the neck exercises can be performed sitting or standing, whichever is more comfortable for you.

FLEXION

While standing, look down and bend your chin forward to your chest. If you feel stiffness or pain, do not force the movement. Go as far as you can without straining yourself. If your muscle pain worsens with this or any exercise, stop until you have talked to your physician or physical therapist.

EXTENSION

Look up and bend your head back as far as possible without forcing any movement.

LATERAL FLEXION

Tilt your left ear to your left shoulder (but do not raise the shoulder). If you feel pain or resistance, do not force the motion.

Now tilt your right ear to your right shoulder, just as you did for the left ear (see figure 5.3).

ROTATION

Turn to look over your left shoulder. Try to make your chin even with your shoulder. Go as far as is comfortable, but do not force the movement.

Now turn and look over your right shoulder, as with the left.

Neck Isometric Exercises

Neck isometric exercises are more advanced exercises to help strengthen the muscles of the neck, which is most important in

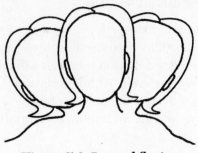

Figure 5.3. Lateral flexion

fibromyalgia. Try these gently and gradually as much as possible after range of motion of your neck is improved. Again, do not hold your breath.

ISOMETRIC FLEXION

1. Place hand on forehead. Try to look down while resisting the motion with your hand. Hold for six seconds, counting out loud.
2. Place your hands on the back of your head. Try to look up and back while resisting the motion with your hands. Hold for six seconds, counting out loud.

ISOMETRIC LATERAL FLEXION

Start with your head straight. Place your left hand just above your left ear (see figure 5.4 on page 111). Try to tilt your head to the left but resist the motion with your left hand. Hold for six seconds, counting out loud.

Now place your right hand just above your right ear. Try to tilt your head to the right but resist the movement with your right hand. Hold for six seconds, counting out loud.

ISOMETRIC ROTATION

Place your left hand above your ear and near your left forehead. Now try to look over your left shoulder, but resist the motion

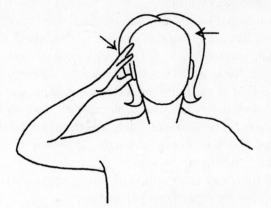

Figure 5.4. Isometric lateral flexion

with your left hand. The hand should not be placed on the jaw. Hold for six seconds, counting out loud.

Now place your right hand above your ear and near your right forehead. Try to look over your right shoulder, but resist the motion with your right hand. Hold for six seconds, counting out loud.

Shoulder Range-of-Motion Exercises

The following five range-of-motion exercises will increase the flexibility of the shoulders and arms. Increasing the number of exercises will increase the strength of the arms.

SHOULDER EXTERNAL ROTATION

This exercise increases the motion you use to comb your hair. You may sit, stand, or lie down to do these exercises.

Clasp your hands behind your head. Pull your elbows together until they are as close as possible in front of your chin. Separate the elbows to the side as much as possible.

Repeat this, gradually increasing to five, then ten, then up to twenty repetitions. You may repeat these two or three times daily.

SHOULDER INTERNAL ROTATION

Shoulder internal rotation increases the flexibility of the shoulders. Using the same motions women use to fasten a bra in the back or men use to put a wallet in a back pocket, move your arms behind your back, as shown in figure 5.5 (see page 113). This exercise is best done standing and is often done in the shower using a washcloth to wash your upper back and a towel to dry it.

Put your hand behind your back, and then put the other hand behind your back and cross the wrist as shown in the picture. Return the hands to rest at your side.

Repeat this twice daily, gradually increasing to five, then ten, then up to twenty repetitions per session.

SHOULDER FLEXION

Shoulder flexion holds both arms down at your sides. Raise the left arm straight up and reach overhead toward the ceiling. Now do the same with the right arm. Continue this motion as you alternate left-right-left-right.

Repeat twice daily, gradually increasing to five, then ten, then up to twenty repetitions per session.

SHOULDER ABDUCTION

Raise both arms straight out away from your sides, and then raise each arm overhead toward the ceiling and up above your head. It doesn't matter whether you do this palm-up or palm-down.

If it's painful to do this exercise while sitting or standing, you can also do it lying on your bed, using a stick (a broom handle will do). As you raise your arms, hold the stick with both hands and keep your arms straight, up over your head as far as possible. The strength of the less painful arm will help the painful arm move more easily.

Repeat this exercise, gradually increasing to five, then ten, then twenty repetitions, two or three times a day.

Once you have mastered the exercise, go to part two of this exercise, which involves raising your arms out to your side, one at a time, then making big circles slowly.

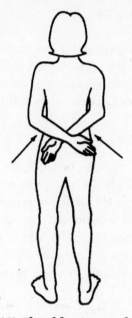

Figure 5.5. Shoulder internal rotation

Repeat this exercise, gradually increasing to five, then ten, then twenty repetitions, two or three times a day.

SHOULDER GIRDLE ROTATION

This exercise can be done in a sitting or standing position and is fun to do during the day to relieve neck and shoulder tension and maintain shoulder girdle flexibility.

Roll shoulders in a forward circle, and raise shoulders toward the ears in a shrugging motion. Then, roll shoulders back and your chest out, as in a military stance. Lower the shoulders and bring them forward. Think of it as a simple shoulder roll in a circle. Now reverse the process, rolling your shoulder girdle in a backward circle.

Repeat this exercise, gradually increasing to five, then ten, then twenty repetitions two or three times a day, if possible.

Back Exercises

As you do the following strengthening exercises, it is very important that you breathe properly while holding a position. Counting to six out loud will enable you to do this easily. If you experience shortness of breath, stop and talk to your doctor or physical therapist.

CHEEK TO CHEEK

This is a convenient exercise because you can do it anywhere, anytime, and practically in any position. It strengthens the muscles of the buttocks that help support the back and the legs. When sitting, you will actually rise up out of the chair because of the contraction of the muscle groups in the buttocks.

Press your buttocks together and hold for a six-second count. Relax and repeat. Gradually increase up to five, then ten, then twenty repetitions.

PELVIC TILT

This is one of the best exercises you can do to strengthen your abdominal muscles, which in turn help support your back. It will also help tone your stomach muscles. Do this exercise lying on your back in bed or on the floor, whichever is more comfortable.

Relax and raise your arms above our head. Keep your knees bent. Now comes the tricky part! Tighten the muscles of your lower abdomen and your buttocks at the same time to flatten your back against the floor or bed. Hold the flat back position for a six-second count. Now relax and repeat.

Repeat this exercise two or three times to start and work gradually to five, then ten, then twenty repetitions twice a day.

If you have trouble, contact your physical therapist or physician and have him or her demonstrate the exercise.

BRIDGING

This exercise strengthens the muscles in the back.

Lie on your back on the floor or in bed and bend your knees. Now lift your hips and buttocks off the bed or floor four to six

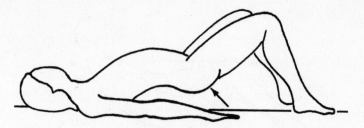

Figure 5.6. A bridging exercise

inches, forcing the small of the back out flat, and tighten the buttock and hip muscles to maintain this position (see figure 5.6 above). Hold this position for a count of six seconds. Relax and lower your hips and buttocks to the floor or bed.

Repeat this exercise, gradually increasing up to five, then ten, then twenty repetitions as tolerated. Repeat twice daily, if possible.

PARTIAL SIT-UP

This is one of the more vigorous exercises. Its purpose is to build abdominal strength, which will give the back greater support. To do this exercise, lie on your bed or on the floor, whichever is more comfortable. Lie on your back with your knees bent. Raise your head and shoulder blades off the floor or bed (see figure 5.7 on page 116). Hold that position for a six-second count. Slowly return to the beginning position. Repeat.

Start this exercise slowly, with one or two repetitions, until your body adjusts. Gradually increase to five, then ten repetitions.

BACK EXTENSION

For this exercise to strengthen the back muscles, lie on your bed or on the floor in a prone (stomach-down) position. A pillow may be used under the stomach to help make this position more comfortable.

Raise your head, arms, and legs off the floor. Do not bend your knees. This must be done with your body straight in extension. Hold for six seconds while you count out loud. Relax and repeat.

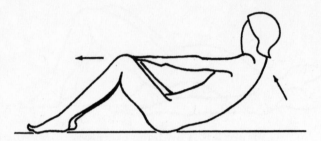

Figure 5.7. A partial sit-up exercise

Gradually increase up to five, then ten repetitions. If you experience discomfort, check with your physician or physical therapist before you continue.

CAT-CAMEL

Do not do this exercise for strengthening the back muscles if you have very painful knees, ankles, or hands, as it places pressure on these areas.

The position for this exercise is a crawling position (see figure 5.8 on page 117). Hands must be directly under your shoulders. Take a deep breath and arch your back as a frightened cat does, lowering your head. Hold that position for six seconds, counting out loud. Now exhale and drop the arched back slowly, raising your head.

Start this exercise slowly with one or two repetitions. Increase up to five and then ten repetitions, if possible.

WALL PUSH

This exercise is good for the back because it encourages the body extension positions.

Stand spread-eagle, with your hands against a wall. Now arch your back inward slowly.

Gradually increase repetitions from one to five, or more. This exercise is fun because you can do it anytime you feel you need a good body stretch. Repeat two times daily.

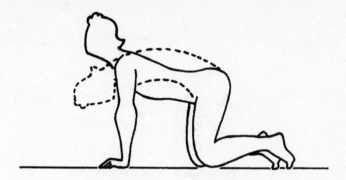

Figure 5.8. A cat-camel exercise

BACK FLEXIBILITY

Lie on your back on the floor with knees bent and feet flat on the floor. Raise hands toward the ceiling. Now move arms and head to the right, while the knees move to the left. Reverse the above, then repeat. Gradually increase up to five and then ten repetitions twice daily.

BICYCLING

Lying on your back, move your feet and legs in the air as if you were riding a bicycle. Count to six and relax. Repeat, then gradually increase to five and then ten repetitions once or twice daily, if tolerated.

Elbow Stretch to Treat Tennis Elbow

With your arm extended straight out, parallel to the floor, lock your elbow and position your palm face up. Using your opposite hand, grab hold of the fingers and pull the palm of the extended hand toward the floor. Hold for ten seconds.

Now do the same but have the palm facing down. Using the opposite hand, push the top of your extended fingers and hand down toward the floor. Hold for ten seconds. Do this stretch several times daily, as needed, for pain and stiffness.

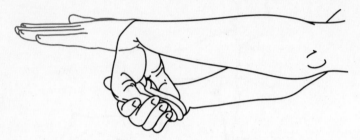

Figure 5.9. Elbow stretch

Endurance or Conditioning Exercises

Recent studies have shown that aerobic fitness is a factor in regulating the altered sleep patterns characteristic of fibromyalgia. Tests have been done on patients, comparing aerobic exercise to range-of-motion or stretching exercises. Although both were found beneficial, patients who performed aerobic exercises regularly showed greater improvement in quality of sleep and trigger-point pain thresholds.

In our clinic, we find that some of the best types of conditioning exercises for patients are walking and water exercises. When performed regularly, these cardiovascular exercises can strengthen muscles and help to relieve depression. And then there's the added benefit of aerobic exercise: It not only challenges the heart and lungs, but by sustaining an elevated heart rate, it will enable you to burn fat and control your weight. Maintaining a normal weight is important for people with any type of chronic pain. It enables you to have more energy and relieves you of unnecessary pressure on painful muscles.

Again, your warm-up should include walking in place for several minutes along with stretching your muscles and joints in full range of motion.

LOW OR HIGH INTENSITY?

When I explained the benefits of exercise in alleviating the deep muscle pain of fibromyalgia to forty-two-year-old Candace, she said there was no way she could ride a bike or run for miles daily. "I can barely walk up the stairs to get in bed each night, much less do endurance exercises."

Many patients who have not exercised for years are overwhelmed by the thought of starting a regular program of physical activity. However, it's important to clarify that regular aerobic exercise does not mean you have to run miles or work up a sweat all the time. Studies show that low-intensity aerobic exercise can give you almost as much benefit over time as high-intensity—and without the risk of injury or exhaustion. This exercise can be walking for thirty to sixty minutes several times a week, swimming laps at the "Y" pool, or walking your dog around the neighborhood after work.

In a controlled trial, exercising twice a week for twenty-five minutes each time, along with two educational sessions, resulted in immediate improvement in patients with fibromyalgia. In another comprehensive study reported in the *Journal of Rheumatology* (March 2002), researchers concluded that high-intensity physical fitness training compared to low-intensity physical fitness training leads to only modest improvements in fitness and well-being in patients with fibromyalgia—and does not positively affect psychological status and general health. I believe studies like these open the door for many who have stayed on the sidelines thinking that unless you were running marathons, you simply weren't exercising hard enough. The truth is out—exercise can be simpler, low intensity, and just as effective in keeping you pain-free and healthy. Choose from the following list of low- to moderate-intensity exercises as you start your program:

FAVORITE ACTIVITIES FOR FMS
Aerobics (low-impact)
Ballroom dancing
Biking

Golf
Hiking
Mall walking
Stair climbing
Stationary cycling
Swimming
Walking
Water exercise

CHECK YOUR PULSE

During exercise, it is important to take your pulse periodically. You can do this by placing your finger (not your thumb) on the artery on the side of your windpipe (your carotid pulse) or on the thumb side of the wrist. Slow your pace during your workout and count your pulse rate for ten seconds. Multiply this number by six to get your total pulse for one minute.

Your pulse rate should stay within your target heart range during exercise. This range can be found using the chart on page 121. Or, you can compute this yourself by subtracting your age from 220 and multiplying the number you get by 60 percent. This gives you the low end of your range. Now subtract your age from 220 and multiply this number by 80 percent to get the high end of your range. If your total pulse rate is higher than your target range, you should slow down. If the pulse rate is lower than the range, you may choose to work harder. Some inactive patients will find that their pulse rate will increase with very little exercise or activity.

The chart provides an estimate for the low and high end of your target heart rate. During exercise, find your pulse rate for one minute as directed. This total rate should fit within the recommended range for safe exercise.

START WITH WALKING

Walking may be the best all-around exercise for people with fibromyalgia. It can be done by almost anyone at any time and at any place . . . and it's free! I've seen patients improve their

ESTIMATED TARGET HEART RANGES FOR VARIOUS AGES DURING EXERCISE

Age	Low	High	Age	Low	High
20–21	120	162	54–55	102	132
22–25	114	156	56–57	96	132
26–27	114	156	58–59	96	126
28–29	114	156	60–62	96	126
30–35	114	150	63–65	96	126
36	108	150	66	90	126
37–44	108	144	67–70	90	120
45	108	138	71–74	90	120
46–51	102	138	75	90	114
52–53	102	132	76–78	84	114

symptoms of pain, stiffness, and fatigue by simply adding fifteen to twenty minutes of walking to their daily routine. Because this low-impact form of exercise is less likely to cause an injury than running or aerobics, it is preferred by many as a safe way to become conditioned.

Beatrice, a forty-four-year-old woman who has lived with fibromyalgia for seven years, said that walking boosts her spirits, especially on days when pain and fatigue seem to overwhelm her. "I love to walk and hike in our neighborhood," she said. "On really bad days when my symptoms flair, I make myself walk anyway. I take a cane to give me added support and allow more time."

Not only will walking tone the muscles in your legs and upper body, but it will increase your metabolism and help with weight management. For women, walking offers a much needed bonus, as it increases bone density, which helps prevent a common disease of aging, *osteoporosis* (brittle bones).

You may wonder about those patients who can barely stand up, much less begin a walking program. In my experience, most people can start this program by making small goals. For example, if you have great pain during movement, begin by walking indoors from room to room for five minutes. As you progress in strength, walk around your house or apartment; then walk around your block. Your pace will depend on your capability and pain threshold, but by taking small steps, most people can achieve an adequate level of fitness. Remember, walking some is better than not walking at all.

Many prefer an indoor treadmill that can be used at home, so bad weather is no excuse, and it can be done anytime, day or night.

REFRESH WITH WATER EXERCISES

Perhaps more than any other conditioning exercise, my patients tell of enjoying water exercises the most. Forty-one-year-old Robert said that water exercise is almost as refreshing as a nap. "I can be having a rough day, feeling sorry for myself and aching all over, then I go over to the swimming pool at my apartment complex and get in the water. Something magical happens while exercising. In just minutes, I feel more optimistic and less pain. It works wonders for me and even helps me to sleep more soundly."

Numerous studies have been done recently on the benefits of water exercise to people with arthritic diseases. The findings are consistent with what Robert claims, that is, water exercise is a perfect no-impact activity that just about anyone can do without injury or stress to an aching joint. Most people report feeling better after a water exercise routine. Stretching or even walking in water is particularly comforting as the buoyancy of the water supports your body, putting less pressure on trigger points.

There are water vests and life jackets you can purchase that allow you to exercise in water without fear of going under. An aqua vest will place you in a near weightless position so you can stretch and strengthen muscles easily.

Most YMCA programs offer aquatic classes, teaching you the range-of-motion and aerobic exercises that can be done in water. Often, special classes are offered specifically for people with arthritis, and the trained instructors can assist you in designing a water exercise program for your specific fibromyalgia needs.

DAILY LIVING ACTIVITIES

Exercise experts are becoming more convinced that daily living activities and household chores such as mopping floors, washing windows, mowing the yard, and heavy gardening are all beneficial when it comes to fitness. When you do these activities, make sure you stretch your muscles so it can be considered a viable workout. Consider adding the following chores and activities as you plan your daily exercise regimen:

Carrying bags of groceries
Gardening
Hiding your remote control and getting up to change
    channels on the TV
Housecleaning
Mopping floors
Parking farther away from the shops at the mall
Playing actively with your kids or grandkids
Raking leaves
Vacuuming
Walking to the bus stop or store
Washing windows

Ancient Disciplines Heal Mind, Body, and Spirit

TRY YOGA TO DE-STRESS AND BECOME FLEXIBLE

Yoga can be a useful tool to help relieve fibromyalgia pain as well as the associated anxiety, depression, and sleep problems. The various postures help to increase flexibility and strength, encourage deep breathing and relaxation, and help you to get in touch with your body, mind, and spirit. There are two studies on osteoarthritis of the hands and carpal tunnel and the practice of yoga; both report greater reduction in pain than in the control groups. Because yoga improves muscle strength and involves stretching and relaxation postures, it should be very advantageous for those with fibromyalgia and other musculoskeletal problems.

Many different styles of yoga are currently being taught. For instance, the gentle practice of Viniyoga, incorporating deep breathing with gentle stretching, is a great way to enhance your health and well-being. The Iyengar style of yoga can help those who are interested in a more intense physical yoga practice to become stronger and reduce chronic pain. With all types of yoga, it is important to find a qualified instructor, one who is knowledgeable about the symptoms and challenges that those with fibromyalgia and deep muscle pain might experience.

YOGA FOCUSES ON MIND-BODY INTERPLAY

Yoga incorporates many elements with the goal of improving your overall health. In ancient India, the yoga sages were interested in helping people to feel whole and spiritually connected. Thus, yoga incorporates physical exercises, as well as moral and ethical codes, concentration exercises, and meditation. You might benefit most from the physical postures (*asanas*) to alleviate aches and pains, concentration exercises (*dharana*) to overcome fibro fog, and meditation (*dhyana*) to help you focus on the present instead of ruminating about daily worries.

PHYSICAL POSTURES (*ASANAS*) RELIEVE PAIN

The physical postures are very helpful if you experience sore muscles on a daily basis. Daily stretching helps to lubricate the joints and sends nutrients and oxygen to the muscles, bathing them in fresh blood. Taking time to relax and enjoy stretching helps to reduce your blood pressure and relieves stress. Especially with the additional stressor of chronic pain, yoga may help you to relieve symptoms of fibromyalgia and cut back on the medication you take.

CONCENTRATION EXERCISES (*DHARANA*) OVERCOME FIBRO FOG

I realize that the experience of chronic pain and insomnia is distressing to many. Not only is it difficult to get through the day without feeling irritable and tired, but also sometimes it's hard not to resent being in this position altogether. In yoga, there are exercises of concentration and meditation that help you to control your thoughts, and to ease the racing thoughts of anxiety and depression. For instance, certain balancing postures like the Tree pose (see page 127) not only improve your physical balance but also help to calm your mind. As one patient, Rosa, said when she started a yoga class for beginners, "It's practically impossible to worry and do these poses at the same time!"

Yoga stretches can help to induce sleep. If you are keyed up prior to bedtime, try the Child's or Corpse pose (see pages 126 and 130). These poses are very calming, and help relax the body and mind. In addition, yoga can help reduce stress and balance moods, which will lessen the severity of the pain you feel.

MEDITATION (*DHYANA*) HELPS YOU TO FOCUS ON THE MOMENT

Meditation is helpful as you clear your mind of racing thoughts and focus on a renewed sense of peace, relaxation, and bliss. Practicing meditation can help ease anxiety and depression by helping you to focus on the moment instead of ruminating on myriad worries and fears. Instead of giving in to negative thoughts, you learn to "feel the breath" and calm the mind to achieve feelings of inner peace. Regular practice of meditation can teach you how to stop anxious feelings before they become full-blown panic attacks. Many yogis feel we hold emotions deep in the body with the outward signs of hunched shoulders, tight lips, and furrowed brows. Through yoga, we can tap into these patterns of chronic tightness, release the muscles, and begin to heal the emotional wounds.

For those struggling with depression or other serious mood disorders, yoga can be an effective addition to regular psychotherapy. While it is recommended that you find an experienced yoga teacher, there are simple yoga exercises that can be done at home with little to no risk of injury. Remember to be aware of your breath as you practice, taking deep, slow inhales and full, complete exhales. The practice of exhaling completely helps to rid the body of toxins and aids in relaxation. Here's a stress-reduction technique that I share with patients: Buy a bottle of inexpensive children's bubbles (in the toy section at any store), and use these to learn how to breathe slowly and evenly. Blow through the bubble blower with a steady stream of breath. If you blow too hard or too softly, you won't get any bubbles. However, you will find that smooth and steady breaths will produce a nice flow of bubbles. Use this breathing technique without the bubbles when you are feeling stressed. Also practice it with the following yoga poses and you'll experience a decrease in the stress response and feel more alert.

CHILD'S POSE

This pose can be done several times a day, as needed, to help calm you down. Kneel on the floor on your hands and knees. Your hands should be under the shoulders and your knees under the hips with toes touching. Stretch your neck forward and lengthen your spine through the tailbone. Gently rock the weight of your body back toward your feet, letting your hips stretch farther back as you continue to lengthen and stretch your spine. Stretch your arms forward and walk your fingertips as far forward as they will go on the floor or rug, lengthening your arms fully. Stretch from the shoulders. As your hips stretch backward, focus on the stretch from the armpits to the hips, lengthening the sides of the torso and the back. If you are flexible, continue stretching and relax your neck as the forehead touches the floor. Pressing the forehead against the floor or pillows helps to calm the mind as the forehead and eye muscles completely relax. If this is hard, put one or two pillows under your forehead.

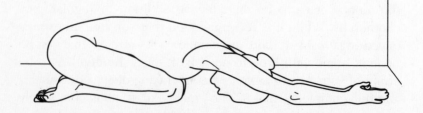

Figure 5.10. Child's pose

Rest a few seconds, allowing the forehead and eye muscles to relax. Let the breath soothe you during this pose. This is a great posture to practice as you prepare for sleep, or if you need a calming moment in a stressful day.

TREE POSE

This pose is great for improving concentration and practicing meditation, and also gives the added benefit of building strength and improving balance. Stand with your side next to a wall. Or use a chair for balance, if you find it difficult to stand on one foot. Stand up straight with big toes touching. Spread the soles of the

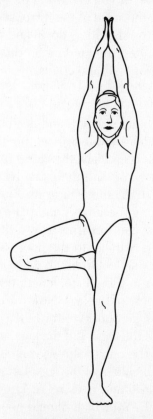

Figure 5.11. Tree pose

feet and feel the whole bottom of the feet supporting your weight. Spread the toes wide and engage the leg muscles so the legs feel strong. Rotate the right hip and knee outward so the right knee points to the right wall. The left knee and foot point forward. Lift the right leg and place the sole of the foot on the inner left leg. You can place the foot on the inner ankle, knee, or thigh, depending on your flexibility. Keep the left leg strong and straight, like a tree trunk. Hold the posture and breathe, keeping the mind calm. If you find it easy to balance on one leg, raise the arms overhead. Continue to keep the left leg strong as you straighten your arms and reach upward toward the sky. Your palms can face each other, or you can bring the palms together. As you reach up, stretch the sides of the torso, keeping the back straight and long. Relax the shoulders down and try not to tense the neck and shoulders. Repeat standing on the right leg, with the left leg raised. Hold for several seconds.

MODIFIED DOG POSE

This easy pose helps to build strength and flexibility and can be done anywhere. Stand facing a wall. Spread the soles of the feet and the toes wide for balance. Place the palms of your hands on the wall in front of your waist, and then step back two or three feet, bend forward, and straighten your arms. Press into the wall with your hands, spreading the fingers and palms wide. Engage the hand muscles, wrists, and forearms as you do so. Your back and spine should now be parallel to the floor. Stretch the tailbone away from the wall, and lengthen the sides of the torso from the armpits to the hips. You should feel length through the arms and torso. Engage the backs of the legs. Now press the heels into the floor and lift the hips (sit bones) toward the ceiling, feeling a nice stretch in the back of the legs. Lift the knee muscles into the quadriceps, and engage the quadriceps as you continue stretching the hamstrings and the backs of the legs. Lengthen the arms, torso, and legs, as the head and neck relax. Lengthen the neck and release it comfortably. Your body should make a right angle to the wall. This pose is great for relieving back and neck pain.

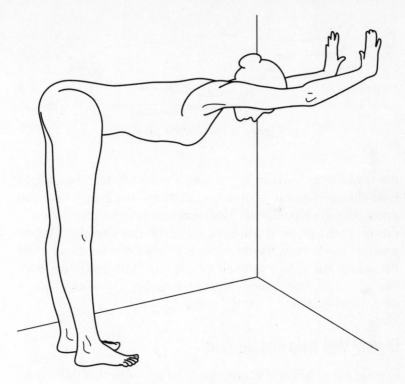

Figure 5.12. Modified dog pose

CORPSE POSE

This relaxing pose is a great way to practice meditation. Lie on your back on a comfortable surface, and stretch your arms and legs out straight. Keep your arms down by your sides, and extend your legs straight from the hips. Your feet should be about twelve inches apart, with both feet turned out slightly to keep the feet, ankles, and legs relaxed. With palms facing upward, keep the arms eight to ten inches from the body. Lengthen the back on the floor and feel all muscles stretching and releasing. Notice your shoulder blades and hips, and adjust the body until you feel balanced on both the left and right sides of the body. Scan your body and consciously relax every muscle group, including the throat, face, and eye muscles. Continue this scanning as you lie

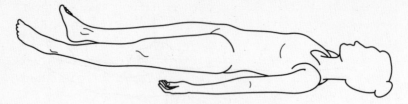

Figure 5.13. Corpse pose

down and relax, and become aware of areas in which you might hold chronic tension. As you lie there, feel the breath take you into a deeper relaxed state. The more you practice meditation in this pose, the easier it will become to still the thoughts. As you practice meditation, do not criticize yourself if you cannot quiet the mind, just accept yourself as you are. With time, the practice of meditation becomes more calming and you will feel more rejuvenated.

Qigong May Help Reduce Pain

Qigong is an ancient Chinese exercise technique that dates back three thousand to five thousand years. Combining meditation with dance, movement, and breathing exercises, qigong helps to improve the body's energy and powers of self-healing. It is said to increase energy, decrease fatigue, and alleviate pain—all of which would be helpful to those with fibromyalgia. Called the "mother of Chinese healing," qigong (pronounced *chee-gong*) is possibly one of the most powerful healing traditions ever developed in human history.

Researchers in the complementary medicine program at University of Maryland School of Medicine in Baltimore are now doing studies on fibromyalgia patients using a combination of qigong; mindfulness meditation, a simple form of meditation from the Buddhist tradition that focuses on awareness of the present moment; and cognitive behavioral therapy. In a previous pilot study at University of Maryland School of Medicine, investigators found that fibromyalgia patients had significant reduction in pain, fatigue, and sleeplessness, and improved mood and functioning, using the combined techniques.

Initially, you may have to pay a practitioner to teach you qigong, or you can sign up for a course at your local community center. There are also instructional videos available in all levels. Once you understand the positions, you can do qigong at any time at no cost. Those who regularly use qigong tell of needing less medication and faster healing. However, the postures or exercises should be done each morning to "build chi." To find a qualified instructor, contact the National Qigong (Chi Kung) Association (see Resources, page 289).

Tai Chi Increases Range of Motion

Tai chi, a form of qigong, may be the perfect exercise for fibromyalgia sufferers as you strive to cope with daily muscle tension, as well as life's stressors. This ancient discipline emphasizes relaxation and passive concentration without risk of injury. Some have even said that it's like "meditation in motion," with dramatic, flowing movements instead of forceful actions. The ultimate goal of tai chi is to bring the principles of yin and yang into natural harmony.

For those who find exercise painful, tai chi may enable you to slowly move your body in a full range of motion, building strength while also receiving the benefit of stress reduction. There are books on tai chi along with videos that you can purchase at online or local bookstores for use in the privacy of your home.

Strengthening Exercises

For those over the age of forty the muscle pain and weakness associated with fibromyalgia present an even greater problem. Studies show that muscle strength naturally levels off at midlife. There is good news, though; resistance or weight training can offset this muscle decline and help build strength in aching muscles.

There used to be hesitation when recommending strength training for those with pain-related ailments like fibromyalgia. Experts felt that strength training would exacerbate fibromyalgia symptoms or cause injury to the muscles or joints. We now know differently, and new studies are confirming that strength training actually increases conditioning, muscle strength, and endurance—as well as alleviates pain, stiffness, fatigue, and depression. One particular study published in *Arthritis Care and Research* (February 2002) concluded that along with aerobic activity, strength training—using hand weights, machines, and the body's own resistance—should be a regular part of a fibromyalgia patient's workout regimen for optimal healing.

Over the past decades, a greater emphasis has been placed on aerobics than weight training for pain relief. However, aerobics is a conditioning exercise for the heart and is not designed for developing muscle size. I have seen many patients become discouraged when, after weeks of aerobic exercise, they don't feel any lessening in deep muscle pain. That is why in order to strengthen your muscles, it is important to supplement your exercise routine.

COMMON MISCONCEPTIONS OF WEIGHT TRAINING

"I don't want to look like a football player," one petite woman said after we set her up with a qualified personal trainer to help with a resistance training program. Many people still associate weights with building bulky muscles, but this is not the case. Let's look at some of the common misconceptions of weight training.

1. **Weight lifting is dangerous.** False. If done with proper technique, lifting weights is a very safe way to tone the body.
2. **If you stop, muscles will turn to fat.** False. This is physiologically impossible. If you stop weight lifting, the muscles will lose size and tone, but only extra calories can be deposited as fat. Resistance training does help you to lose weight by replacing fat with lean muscles. While fat burns 2 to 3 calories per pound, muscle burns 50 calories per

pound. The more muscle mass your body has, the more calories you burn all day, even while you are sitting around.

3. **Women will get big muscles.** False. Women produce less testosterone than men and build muscle size less rapidly. It takes years of hard work and proper diet to obtain large muscles.

4. **Strength training means using heavy equipment.** False. Resistance bands can be used as strength training. Other ways to strength-train include using isometrics, free weights, or even water-resistant exercises.

5. **You must start with heavy weights.** False. You should *not* begin with heavy weights. A good rule is to start with a weight you can easily lift ten times with the last two repetitions being increasingly difficult. For some people this is only one to two pounds; others can start at fifteen to twenty pounds, depending on their muscle strength. As your muscles gain strength and if there is no pain, increase the weights in one- to two-pound increments.

6. **The theory "no pain, no gain" is true for strength training.** False. If your muscles are very sore, do not use resistance training until you are relatively pain-free. Strength training may not be appropriate for every patient; check with your doctor for approval.

7. **You will get high blood pressure.** False. Weight training does not cause high blood pressure. Some people strain their body and hold their breath during a lift, which results in a temporary increase of blood pressure. However, holding your breath is *never recommended* during weight training.

8. **You will become bulky and inflexible.** False. It is important to supplement your weight training with a stretching routine to stay flexible. As an added bonus, resistance training may have a more lasting effect on metabolism than aerobic exercise. It burns fat and increases muscle mass. Resistance training also elevates metabolism for up to two hours after you finish the workout.

9. **Lifting weights helps you spot-reduce specific areas of your body.** False. Exercise is not site-specific; you must exercise the total body to achieve maximum results.
10. **The benefits are many.** True. Increased strength, improved muscle tone, enhanced athletic performance, increased bone, tendon, and ligament strength, injury prevention, and improved body image are all benefits of weight training. For women, weight training can play a significant role in preventing osteoporosis, as bones need regular resistance to stay strong. And age is no factor with weight training; the muscles of older people can be responsive to training.

GETTING STARTED WITH WEIGHT TRAINING

As you plan your resistance program, you should lift at least two to three times per week, with at least forty-eight to seventy-two hours between sessions for muscles to recover. Select an exercise for each of the body parts: legs (calves, quads, and hamstrings), abdomen, back, chest, shoulders, and arms (biceps and triceps).

One problem with weight training: Neglecting to exercise a body part can lead to imbalances in your body. Proper form is critical, whether you use free weights or machines. To ensure proper form and technique, it would be advantageous to use a qualified personal trainer the first few sessions. Your physician can help you find a trainer, if needed.

Initially, you should start out using very light weights or resistance of only one to two pounds, concentrating more on form. Gradually add weight and maintain proper form. Once you find a comfortable weight, you should stay with it for one to two sets of ten repetitions per body part, taking one to three minutes between sets to ensure a good-quality workout.

TRY CIRCUIT TRAINING

Another way to weight-train is called circuit training. This is a group of machines that exercises all the body parts. You may be less likely to get injured using machines than using free weights.

Free weights also can take months of practice before you become adept at sophisticated lifting techniques.

NO TIME TO EXERCISE?

Many patients claim they'd be more likely to exercise if there were more hours in the day. Well, we cannot change time, so let me suggest a workable alternative: divide your exercise workout into three 10-minute segments, what I call "mini-bursts." These mini-bursts of exercise are known to give excellent cardiovascular benefit, as well as keep your muscles fit, your joints mobile, and your body slim, as you burn calories to maintain a normal weight. Perhaps the greatest benefit of mini-bursts is seen in mood and energy levels. Researchers from Northern Arizona University found that just ten minutes of pedaling on a stationary bike was all that was necessary to improve overall mood and banish fatigue. Now add a brisk ten-minute walk at lunchtime and ten minutes of low-impact aerobics after dinner, and you've done a lot to improve your physical and mental conditioning.

SUGGESTED 10-MINUTE MINI-BURSTS
10-minute walk before work
10-minute walk at the mall before you shop
10-minute ride on the stationary bike during the noon news
10-minute walk on your indoor treadmill
10-minute swim in the neighbor's pool
10-minute bike ride with your child after school
10-minute walk around the block
10 minutes of low-impact aerobics using a videotape

SEVEN DAYS TO END PAIN

The following plan will help you halt or even reverse the pain you feel each day, as well as ease muscle tension and increase deep sleep. Once you've done the initial seven days, repeat the schedule, slowly increasing exercise and activity if you can. Even if you only do half the suggested exercises the first week, I want you to get started. I've had patients start out with five minutes of walking every other day. They'd tell me how much it hurt and how difficult it was to start, but within six months, these same patients were walking several miles a day. They stuck with the commitment to exercise, and they slowly conditioned their body and became physically fit over a period of months. As I promised these patients, I will make the same pledge to you: The more active you become, the less pain you will feel. You will sleep better, have fewer mood swings, and have a more positive outlook on life. Be sure to talk with your doctor before doing these exercises and stay on prescribed medications.

Day	Time of Day	Action
Day 1:	7:00 A.M.	Moist heat for 15 minutes
	7:15 A.M.	Stretching and range-of-motion exercises (5 minutes)
	7:20 A.M.	Walk or use stationary bike (10 minutes)
	7:30 P.M.	Moist heat for 15 minutes
	8:00 P.M.	Stretching and range-of-motion exercises (5 minutes)
Day 2	7:00 A.M.	Moist heat for 15 minutes
	7:15 A.M.	Stretching and range-of-motion exercises (5 minutes)
	7:20 A.M.	Resistance training (free weights; 10 minutes)
	7:30 P.M.	Moist heat for 15 minutes
	7:45 P.M.	Stretching and range-of-motion exercises (5 minutes)
Day 3	7:00 A.M.	Moist heat for 15 minutes
	7:15 A.M.	Stretching and range-of-motion exercises (10 minutes)
	7:25 A.M.	Stationary bicycle (10 minutes)
	7:30 P.M.	Moist heat for 15 minutes
	7:45 P.M.	Yoga postures (10 minutes)

Day	Time of Day	Action
Day 4	7:00 A.M.	Moist heat for 15 minutes
	7:15 A.M.	Stretching and range-of-motion exercises (10 minutes)
	7:25 A.M.	Resistance training (free weights; 15 minutes)
	7:30 P.M.	Moist heat for 15 minutes
	7:45 P.M.	Repeat morning exercises and light stretching
Day 5	7:00 A.M.	Moist heat for 15 minutes
	7:15 A.M.	Stretching and range-of-motion exercises (15 minutes)
	7:30 A.M.	Swim (10 minutes)
	7:30 P.M.	Moist heat for 15 minutes
	7:45 P.M.	Yoga postures
Day 6	7:00 A.M.	Moist heat for 15 minutes
	7:15 A.M.	Stretching and range-of-motion exercises (10 minutes)
	7:30 A.M.	Resistance training (15 minutes)
	7:30 P.M.	Moist heat for 15 minutes
	7:45 P.M.	Stretching and range-of-motion exercises (10 minutes)
Day 7	7:00 A.M.	Moist heat for 15 minutes
	7:15 A.M.	Stretching and range-of-motion exercises (10 minutes)
	7:30 A.M.	Walk (15 minutes)
	7:30 P.M.	Moist heat for 15 minutes
	7:45 P.M.	Yoga postures (10 minutes)

Heat or Ice?

All of the exercises described in this chapter will be much more effective and you will be more comfortable doing them if, before beginning, you take a warm shower for five to ten minutes to help you loosen up. You can even begin stretching while in the shower. After you complete the exercise program, take another warm shower if you have pain.

Some people feel more relief when they use ice packs instead of moist heat. A plastic bag or ice bag filled with ice can be applied to the painful area for about ten minutes. Don't place ice directly on your skin. Some patients get the most relief when they alternate treatments—moist heat then ice pack. Choose the combination that works best for you.

Remember—those who do their exercises regularly have a much higher chance of improving their symptoms. Do your exercises on good days and bad days, even when it is inconvenient. Once you are used to exercising, the time needed will be minimal and the rewards will be great. People frequently tell me that when they do their exercises they feel much better—and when they skip them, they feel worse. Exercises work!

Exercise Cautions for Fibromyalgia Patients

Although an ongoing, daily exercise program will help you to see the short-term results of increased mobility and decreased pain, it can take months to build strong muscles. You can make the muscles that support your aching joints stronger and more flexible, but it takes time.

It is important to set personal exercise goals as you begin the prevention plan. Your goal may be to exercise for five minutes each day for the first two weeks. Once you get into the habit of doing this, then increase this exercise goal by another five minutes until you reach the suggested fifteen to twenty minutes or more of conditioning exercises, four to five times a week. Be sure you include a warm-up (walking or light jogging in place) before you begin your workout, then move to stretching, conditioning, and a few minutes of cooldown, which can include walking around while stretching your muscles again.

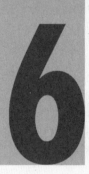

STEP 3:
DE-STRESS YOUR LIFE

"Doctor, I do apologize for being here, for I know you think I'm crazy." If I've heard this statement once, I've heard it hundreds of times. The varying, nonspecific symptoms of fibromyalgia, along with no scientific means to diagnose the disease, makes it is easy to feel as if the condition is imagined or in one's head. But research has shown again and again that fibromyalgia is not a psychiatric illness, even though millions of fibromyalgia patients have psychiatric symptoms, including depression, anxiety, and related disorders.

There is great speculation that stress or an inability to handle life's daily stressors may play an important part in the ebb and flow of fibromyalgia symptoms. Some researchers have tried to correlate high levels of stress with susceptibility to viral infection, whereas others have speculated that fibromyalgia could be viewed as "associated with dysregulation of the stress system."

If you are like many of my patients with fibromyalgia, perhaps you need to know how to de-stress your life so that these additional symptoms don't become a permanent fixture. Brenda, a middle-aged mother of teenage sons, tells of feeling nervous and having frequent panic attacks, especially when her fibromyalgia symptoms flair. But it may not be the fibromyalgia that is causing this excess anxiety; Brenda also tells of being "on call" for everyone in her family in addition to working part-time and caring for her aging parents.

Brenda's enslavement to pleasing those around her without thought of her own health and well-being is shared by many today, especially women. It can cause problems when you have a chronic disease and are faced with a new set of limitations. Fortunately, these limitations can be lessened if you take active steps to get your life and priorities in order.

Is There a Fibromyalgia Personality?

Although in the past, some observations have described a stereotypical obsessive-compulsive, perfectionistic fibromyalgia personality, current studies do not support this observation. Using standard diagnostic criteria, researchers found that only 5 to 6 percent of fibromyalgia patients could be classified as having obsessive-compulsive disorder (OCD). Using psychological testing, these researchers found that approximately one-third of fibromyalgia patients are psychologically fragile, one-third have a chronic pain profile, and one-third are "normal."

It is important to understand that patients with fibromyalgia will always score high on the hypochondriasis and hysteria scales of these tests, since such scales are scored by summing the patient's physical complaints. It makes sense that if a well person were in constant pain and could not achieve restful sleep because of fibromyalgia, her complaints might also be magnified and appear to be psychological in nature.

It's important to note that pain is more than an unpleasant physical "feeling." It is also an emotional experience that makes you irritable, anxious, and depressed. Chronic pain can leave you feeling hopeless. When your life is disrupted with pain, every facet of your existence is affected. While there is still some controversy regarding fibromyalgia and psychological problems, I have seen that when patients reduce stress in their lives, they also experience a reduction in depression, anxiety, and fatigue, as sleep becomes more restful. Because they feel more in control, the symptoms that were once immobilizing subside and quality of life is realized.

The Mind-Body Interplay

In simplest terms, stress is a response of the body to any demand. It is a biological phenomenon that affects both the central and autonomic nervous systems, as well as the endocrine and immune systems. And it is a key contributing factor to illness, including heart disease, depression, anxiety disorders, asthma and allergy, cancer, and even fibromyalgia.

While there is still some controversy regarding the role of stress in fibromyalgia, there are theories that suggest that it is the annoying daily hassles, not major life stressors, that greatly affect these patients and their symptoms. Especially when coupled with low levels of support from family, friends, coworkers, and even personal physicians, psychological stress may increase the patient's reaction to pain and escalate the chances that pain will occupy her attention. Some theorize that those with fibromyalgia experience higher levels of life stress and lower levels of social support than do healthy individuals.

Evaluate Your Stress Level

How often do you feel stressed? Some patients tell of feeling too much stress during the time when their symptoms flare. On the other hand, many fibromyalgia patients admit that they feel stressed every minute of every day. A recent survey found that 16 percent of those questioned felt stressed "all the time" and could not seem to relax, not even for a minute, while 52 percent of those questioned felt stressed "most of the time."

Every week an estimated 95 million Americans suffer a stress-related problem and take medication for their aches and pains. There are estimates that as much as 80 percent of all illness is stress-related, and 85 percent of all industrial accidents are linked to personal worker behavior that includes adaptation to stress. In new data from a study done by the Massachusetts Institute of Technology Analysis Group, researchers estimate that depression, which can be triggered by ongoing stress, costs American business $43.7 billion a year—as much as heart disease.

Study after study indicates that stress is skyrocketing, so you'd better fasten your seat belt, because there is no indication that stress will level off anytime soon. In fact, many people report that they are *more stressed* now than five or ten years ago. As Kim, a thirty-eight-year-old high school English teacher, said, "I get high anxiety just lying in bed thinking about what I have to do at school that day. Imagine how I feel at the end of my day!"

You don't have to imagine how Kim feels because you've probably been there. You know how stress makes your fibromyalgia symptoms worsen. Yet have you identified the areas in your life that are harried, hurried, and out of control?

Check each of the following problems or life interruptions that may negatively affect your body, and then use the suggestions in this chapter to make positive lifestyle changes.

___ too little sleep
___ too much sleep
___ negative attitude
___ hostility
___ depression
___ repressed feelings
___ sense of worthlessness
___ inability to communicate
___ poor diet
___ very little exercise
___ loneliness
___ recent job loss or lack of employment
___ job dissatisfaction
___ recent death of a loved one
___ caregiving to a chronically ill person
___ marital separation and/or divorce
___ exposure to environmental pollutants

__ smoking
__ heavy alcohol use
__ long-term medication usage

Because stress can show itself through a wide variety of physical changes and emotional responses in fibromyalgia, it is important to identify what causes these feelings. Stress symptoms vary greatly from one person to the next, and learning to identify the ways in which your body and mind show stress is an important step in treating and managing this disease.

THE SYMPTOMS OF STRESS
Anger
Anxiety
Back pain
Body aches and pains
Boredom
Bossiness
Change in bowel or bladder habits
Compulsive eating or gum chewing
Constant worrying
Crying
Dizziness
Dry mouth
Feeling of doom
Forgetfulness
Headaches and other aches
Inability to make decisions
Increased usage of drugs, alcohol, or cigarettes
Indigestion
Lack of creativity
Light-headedness
Loneliness
Loss of sense of humor
Memory loss
Palpitations

Racing heart
Restlessness
Ringing in ears
Sleep problems
Sweaty palms
Teeth grinding
Unhappiness

Not All Stress Is Harmful

Stress can be viewed as positive or negative, and the way we interpret the stress creates differences in our personal responses. In the past decade, research in the field of psycho-neuroimmunology (PNI) has shown that life's stressors can produce the same initial physical response of adrenaline rush whether the stress is perceived as positive or negative. For example, you may cringe at the thought of skydiving, whereas your best friend would push to be first in line. Receiving an award and giving an acceptance speech might be considered exciting for one person, whereas even the thought of being in the spotlight might make another person visibly ill.

This observation also applies to those with fibromyalgia. I've had some patients who wake up anxious about what lies ahead of them, even when their day does not appear to be stressful. Louise told of how she would lie awake at night and anticipate how horrible she was going to feel the next day. "When the alarm goes off, I feel like crying. I'm tired from lack of sleep, my body aches, and I dread starting a new day," she said.

Yet other patients see each day as an opportunity, no matter what their pain or fatigue threshold is at that particular time. Raymond, a forty-one-year-old tax attorney, was diagnosed with fibromyalgia three years ago, yet he is certainly not waiting for this disease to take over his life. "I've got too much to do," Raymond said. "I've revamped my schedule to rest throughout the day, but other than that, I still do the very activities that I want to. I cannot imagine giving in to the pain and fatigue."

Both good and bad stress can affect fibromyalgia. The roles of perceived stress and psychological factors are controversial in fibromyalgia studies. Many reports show that patients report a heightened awareness of symptoms when facing stress, whether good or bad.

Good stress, or eustress. Positive stress, or *eustress,* still signals the fight-or-flight response as does negative stress, but this adrenaline high usually gives us the energy to enjoy the moment. Positive stressors, such as a promotion or buying a new home, have been linked with increased productivity, happiness, and longevity. Yet for the person with a chronic disease, such as fibromyalgia, these positive events can also be interpreted in a negative manner. As one new grandmother told me, "Just thinking about traveling to take care of my new grandbaby makes me anxious and fatigued."

Bad stress, or distress. Negative stress, or *distress,* also signals adrenaline to rush through your body, but it is this type of stress that puts you into the full-blown stress response and if continuous can lead to loss of productivity, burnout, and health problems, including a higher risk of getting diseases. For people with fibromyalgia, negative stressors, such as losing one's job or the illness of a loved one, can make symptoms that were controlled become active once again.

Stress and Fibromyalgia

The following list will give you an idea of what can add to your stress level each day:

THE STRESS IN YOUR LIFE
Waiting in long lines of traffic
Not being able to relax
Having fear of rejection from family and friends
Not getting recognized for abilities at work or home

Coping with too much noise at home or work
Going shopping and having to make choices
Having an overall dull feeling
Having to attend a party with friends
Not being able to express self
Not getting enough sleep
Meeting with the boss about a raise
Waking up feeling tired each day
Getting too much sleep and still feeling tired
Going out to dinner with family and friends
Overall tired feeling all day long
Annoying people
Being the guest of honor at a party
Misplacing or losing things
Going shopping with friends
Inability to concentrate at work or at home
Fear of confrontation with coworkers or family members
Entertaining friends at home
Inability to get close to coworkers or friends
Problems filling out forms
Preparing for the holidays
Dislike of preparing meals each day
Raising active children
Redecorating the house
Receiving a compliment from the boss
Having concerns about health and fibromyalgia
Vacation with family
Getting the yard work completed
Having no energy to do housework
Not having enough money to make ends meet
Too many medical bills, and the insurance won't cover all of
    them
Having to wait in line anywhere
Having to wait to see a doctor
Having a doctor not believe that the symptoms are real
Sexual problems with mate

Marital problems
Physical reaction to weather changes
Not enough energy to keep up in life
Declining physical abilities

After perusing the list, you may wonder why there are no major stressors listed, such as death of a loved one. If what current research indicates is true, patients with fibromyalgia are more stressed with daily hassles than they are with major life intrusions. In other words, waiting in a line of traffic or wondering how you are going to do your housework with all the pain and fatigue may cause you more apparent stress than a sudden crisis.

However, whatever your problems with fibromyalgia, too much stress does not have to be one of them. You can learn to manage your reaction to stress just as you do other areas of your life.

Melding the Body and Mind

Not only have scientists explored how stress may weaken the immune system, making us susceptible to diseases, they are also discovering how to meld the body and mind with psychological techniques—techniques that you can easily incorporate into your daily routine to reduce the threat to your immune system and well-being.

The key to reducing the stress that accompanies fibromyalgia lies in recognizing the signs and taking active steps to reduce these before the stress further injures your health and self-esteem. It is not difficult to start the stress-reduction program given in this chapter and incorporate it into your daily lifestyle.

Evaluate Your Commitments

BUDGET YOUR TIME

Do you find that there is never enough time in the day? Setting priorities and budgeting your time each day is the first step in gaining balance in your life, thus eliminating needless stress and anxiety. You can begin to do this by making a list of all of your commitments—family, work, community involvement, friends— and eliminating those commitments that are not absolutely necessary. Especially when you live with chronic pain and fatigue, you must allow for times during the day when you are not at your peak performance. This means not complicating your life with a list of activities and commitments that are just not important.

MAKE TO-DO LISTS DAILY

Write down tasks that face you each day. As you schedule your day, budget ample time to get your work completed by calculating how long it will take to finish each project—then add on an extra fifteen to thirty minutes, to allow yourself to go at a moderate speed instead of in high gear. This will give you leeway, especially on days when pain and fatigue might hold you back from optimum performance.

If you find that you have more tasks scheduled than time available, rewrite your list and prioritize the projects that *must* be done; put the less important projects or activities at the bottom of the list. These can always wait until another day, or you can delegate them to others. Sharing the load is crucial as you learn to balance your day, doing what your body will let you do without excessive pain and fatigue.

Some people prefer to make their to-do lists each morning, while others find that doing it the night before relieves their minds and enables them to sleep soundly.

SCHEDULE YOUR DAY FOR PEAK EFFICIENCY

For those of you who work, staying employed is obviously a major commitment; but working late into the evening hours or seven days a week is something you can—and must—change.

Some people find that stimulation during late afternoon and evening hours makes it even more difficult to experience restful sleep; if you fall into this category, you may want to exclude evening activities. If mornings are your worst time with pain and fatigue, then plan your day around this and make your main commitments, such as business meetings or shopping, during midday or afternoon.

ACCEPT YOUR LIMITATIONS

When Katrina came to see me, she was at the brink of a divorce from her husband of nineteen years. "This disease has ruined my life. Not only have I lost my health, but my marriage is almost over." Through some intense counseling and a greater understanding of fibromyalgia, Katrina and her husband have worked through their marital problems. But first, she had to accept her limitations. Instead of denying the disease's existence and feeling anger and resentment for its symptoms, Katrina has come to accept it as a new part of her life, realizing that it is not terminal and learning to work around the symptoms to do the very things she enjoys.

Many of the fibromyalgia patients I've treated tell of always trying to achieve the best in whatever they do, and researchers are finding that perfectionism may be an identifying factor for those with this disease. A constant push for perfection can cause undue stress, which results in hazards to mental and physical well-being. Make sure that in all you do, the amount of time you put into the activity or job is well worth the end result. If it isn't, back off and let go of the perfectionistic attitude.

Which of the following perfectionistic beliefs motivate you each day?

- I must achieve my best, no matter how badly I feel.
- I cannot accept anything but perfection in all I do, or I criticize myself harshly.
- No matter how hard I try, I never feel like I've done enough or given enough.
- I would rather work at being perfect than spend pleasurable time with family and friends.

To reduce stress associated with fibromyalgia, you must realize that as a human being you are imperfect, even though you are endeavoring to become something more than you are now. Accepting this tension, you can begin to make some changes in your expectations of yourself. These changes can help you relax so that you can enjoy your life and experience a greater sense of well-being.

IDENTIFY YOUR PERSONAL STRESS REACTION

The initial impact of fibromyalgia on someone is always one of increased reactivity. This means that normally you may be able to handle a large workload, but now that you suffer with symptoms like constant fatigue, general feelings of anxiety or sadness, and muscle aches, any extra stress will put you in reactive gear. When we are in reactive gear, we are driven impulsively by our emotions and how we feel. Not only does reactive gear make us feel vulnerable, it can affect our relationships at home and on the job in a negative manner.

Determine how your body responds to additional stress now that you have been diagnosed with fibromyalgia. What are your stress warning signs as shown on pages 143 to 144? By knowing your own specific stress reactions, you can learn to listen to your body before the stress immobilizes you.

IDENTIFY AND REMOVE STRESS

The main strategy in dealing with stress is to identify and remove or reduce the source. If you react to the stress of being overworked, learn to delegate at your office or at home. If your stress is from overextending yourself with outside commitments, rethink how to modify your priorities and put this plan into action. If your stress stems from the fear of going to bed each night knowing that you are going to toss and turn, try to improve this by using the information in chapter 8 to ensure sounder sleep. If your stress is from facing each day knowing that you may have pain and fatigue, plan ahead the night before. For example, if you set out your clothes and get up thirty minutes earlier, you can move slowly without the necessity of hurrying.

As you seek to minimize stress, ask yourself the following:

- What stressors can I eliminate in my life?
- What stressors can I avoid?
- How can I reduce their intensity or manage them?
- What strategies do I need to use to make these changes?

MAKE JOB-SITE MODIFICATIONS

Fibromyalgia patients who are able to work outside the home tell of experiencing great stress on the job. Some tell of fearing they may be let go as healthier and more qualified workers enter the job force, whereas others are concerned that they are not able to perform the way they used to. Employers also tell of being concerned with the output of chronically ill patients, citing reduced productivity, increased absenteeism, poor work quality, and increased rates of on-the-job accidents.

To continue to be a productive employee, you need to stay mentally and physically able to handle your job responsibilities. You may need to allow more time during the day to get your responsibilities completed. Elizabeth told of talking with her employer about her illness and working out a plan that would benefit both. "I realized that I became very tired during midday," she said. "At that time, I was of no use to anyone, so with my boss's consent, I mapped out a plan to get my work completed on these bad days by taking a two-hour lunch break to nap, then staying a bit later to finish my reports. It has worked for both of us."

Other job-site modifications might involve taking work home on days when you feel fatigued or working on a Saturday morning so you can take extra-long lunch breaks during the week to rest. Whatever you do, avoid procrastination. This may give you a break initially, but when it comes time for the work to be completed, you will feel more stress than ever. It has been said that procrastinators are perfectionists just waiting for that perfect time to do their work. Remember, there is no perfect time! Budget your time, follow your daily to-do lists, and limit your outside commitments on workdays.

Other steps for modifying work stress include:

- Ask for help from coworkers on days when pain and fatigue are overwhelming. Pay them back with your assistance on days when you feel better.
- Take periodic breaks to avoid getting overtired or stressed during busy workdays.
- Listen to music during your workday if you can to help keep stress levels low (see chapter 7 for benefits of music therapy).

Coping with work stress requires that you keep things in perspective. Again, this means that you must seek a balance between self, family, community, and work. This will help you maintain a support network to keep you centered and enable you to have strength to get through the day—even when symptoms flair.

INCREASE COMMUNICATION SKILLS

With a chronic disease like fibromyalgia, communication is the most important tool you have to decrease conflict with family, friends, and coworkers, especially when you feel anger or resentment from having unending pain and fatigue. Preoccupation with your illness causes a tremendous amount of distracting mental activity that can hinder productive communication. If you are feeling overwhelmed by the stress of fibromyalgia, you may find it necessary to have psychological counseling to help you develop appropriate and functional communication strategies to deal with your disease and its effect on your life.

Learn to say "no." Failing to set limits or say no to too many demands will put you in overload and add to your already rising stress level. Try to reach any decision that will involve a physical and mental commitment before you are put on the spot. It is much easier to say no to a persuasive friend when you have thought out the situation beforehand and have checked your calendar. Weigh the alternatives of making a new commitment, and include family members or friends in the discussion. Would another commitment prevent you from getting the rest, exercise, and relaxation you need to feel well? Would it take away from those priorities that are foremost on your list?

The desire to help others is commendable. But if being all things to all people is hindering your healing and making you feel resentful, tired, and depressed, it is time to take a firm stand. Say no—and mean it. You will feel physically and emotionally stronger if you make only those commitments that you can keep without undue stress.

Learn to remove yourself emotionally from stressful situations. Sometimes we magnify problems, making them seem far greater than they are. The stress reaction is triggered by our perception. When we imagine something to be a life-and-death situation, our bodies react as if we are in danger, even if no danger exists.

Work at tempering your emotions as problems come up throughout the day. Instead of every crisis being horrible, learn to view life's interruptions as inconvenient but tolerable. You will find that when you see life as something that you can easily handle, it will not overpower you when trouble hits.

Use Ten Techniques to Overcome Fibro Fog and Improve Your Memory

If you cannot remember what you had for dinner last night and your neighbor's last name is on the tip of your tongue but has yet to come to mind, you're definitely not alone. Studies are now conclusive that cognitive impairment in fibromyalgia patients, specifically memory and vocabulary deficiencies, is quite real.

Cognition is necessary to do many daily tasks, including balancing your checkbook or remembering names, phone numbers, and your to-do list.

If the memory glitches associated with fibro fog get you down, there are ten "techniques" I recommend to patients to help them stay focused and reclaim memory.

1. Keep a pad and pen nearby to jot down key information. Writing down dates, grocery items, friends' names or needs, and even thoughts you want to share with your spouse or family will help you to stay focused. Keep your notes in a specific place you will see often, such as on the refrigerator or taped to the desk calendar or your bathroom mirror. Some patients keep daytimers or notebooks with their "valuable information," including their shopping lists, key phone numbers, address book, checkbook, and other pertinent information. Find what works for you—and use it.

2. Focus on what people are saying when you are communicating with others. Try to pay close attention when people speak. You might repeat what they say back to them in a question format, such as, "So you think Justin is the best applicant?" If you really focus on what the person is saying and then repeat the information back, either aloud or to yourself, you will have a better chance of remembering.

3. Use word association. If you can't remember names, connect the person's name with a specific characteristic that describes the person like "Calm Candace" or "Lean Larry."

4. Turn phone numbers into words, if these are hard to recall. For instance, the number 438-263-6679 could become GET-A-MEMORY. Who could forget that one! One of my patients with a large family used this word/number association frequently and said one young adult child's phone number became NAP-O-CAB (627-6222). Of course, the word combination made no sense, but she felt it was easier to remember nonsense words than the combination of numbers. Find the system that works best for you!

5. Organize grocery lists into meaningful categories. If you forget the list, the categories will remind you of specific items. For instance, a grocery list divided into dairy, produce, frozen foods, meats, cereals, breads, and sweets will help you remember which foods you need when you get to those aisles at your store.

6. Use visualization. Try to create a mental image of the thing you need to remember. Concentrate on a color, an animal or object, or something unique to trigger your memory later. For instance, you might think of pure white snow to remind you to buy laundry detergent.

7. Eliminate distractions as much as possible. If you try to remember someone's name or make a list while talking to your child, or have the radio or television blasting, you're more likely to forget something important.

8. Try to keep your office or home organized in a logical way. When things are always kept in the same place, it is easier to remember where they are. When you come in from an outing, put your keys in your purse or on the desk. Do this every time so this becomes mere habit—something you do without thinking.

9. Rely on a kitchen timer to jolt your memory. For instance, if you are supposed to get the clothes out of the dryer in ten minutes, set the timer and let it "think" for you. Or if you need to leave for work at 7:00 A.M., set a timer to remind you of the deadline.

10. Put it to music. Some patients find that singing helps them to remember certain things more easily. For example, you might sing a friend's street address to the tune of "Mary Had a Little Lamb." Or you might sing a reminder to yourself to "pick up the kids after piano lessons at 5:00 P.M."

KEEP A DAILY JOURNAL

Writing in a journal every day can lend itself to great self-inquiry and allow you to experience a higher plane of consciousness—with enhanced awareness, along with the practice of self-discipline.

With any chronic disease, patients often hide or are even unaware of intense feelings of resentment, anger, and loss. The intense self-inquiry process of keeping a journal can open the pathways to discover these destructive inner feelings and deepest concerns. Some patients can even identify a series of events that are associated with the beginning of fibromyalgia symptoms, offering a possible cause of how and when the symptoms began.

Keeping a journal can also assist you in tracking your muscle pain and fatigue and what the cause may be. For example, you may write in your journal that you are having great pain and feeling exhausted after working in your garden for several days. Months later, you can look back on this date and begin to see a pattern between the increase in your fibromyalgia symptoms and possible lifestyle triggers. Perhaps you find that you haven't slept well in days. Looking back over your journal will enable you to see any emotional or physical problems you may have had that contributed to the sleep problem.

ELIMINATE OR REDUCE CAFFEINE INTAKE

Caffeine is one of the few food products that mimics the stress response. Although a little caffeine may make you feel less tired on a bad morning when you've tossed and turned all night, too much can add to your already stressed emotional state, causing a short-term rise in blood pressure and increased heart rate and anxiety levels. Too much caffeine can greatly increase nervousness, which is a problem fibromyalgia patients do *not* need.

As you make plans to de-stress your life, try limiting your amount of caffeine intake, or better still, eliminate it altogether. Tea and chocolate drinks contain caffeine as well, plus ingredients like theophylline and theobromine, which also can stimulate the heart and central nervous system. Watch that chocolate candy bar you may eat, for it contains caffeine, too. I have found that there is no exact level of caffeine that is okay for everyone, so most patients choose to stop using it altogether.

FOODS HIGH IN CAFFEINE

Coffee, drip	5 oz. (90–115 mg)
Coffee, perk	5 oz. (60–125 mg)
Coffee, instant	5 oz. (60–80 mg)
Coffee, decaf	5 oz. (2–5 mg)
Tea, 5-minute steep	5 oz. (40–100 mg)
Tea, 3-minute steep	5 oz. (20–50 mg)
Hot cocoa	5 oz. (2–10 mg)
Cola soft drink	12 oz. (45 mg)
Chocolate bar	2 oz. (30 mg)

USE MIND-BODY TOOLS FOR RELAXATION

There is evidence that a variety of relaxation therapies, including meditation, prayer, music therapy, deep abdominal breathing, biofeedback, and visualization, are useful in reducing stress and stress-related illness.

When you meditate and experience the relaxation response, your body switches from the pumping "fight or flight" response to a calmer, more peaceful mood. Studies show that when you withdraw from problems and use mind-body tools for relaxation, you can produce alpha and theta waves consistent with serenity and happiness (see chapter 7).

VISIT A DAY SPA

I have many FMS patients who regularly go to day spas for healing massages or other relaxing therapies. These mini-spas cater to the busy man or woman who is low on time and high on stress, and they offer an easily accessible and relaxing spa experience. You can find listings of day spas in the Yellow Pages of your phone book. Some day spas focus exclusively on beauty and body treatments; others are located in health clubs or fitness facilities with expanded services that include aerobic exercise classes, toning and conditioning, yoga, and stretching classes.

You might choose to visit the spa ahead of time. You want to make sure it is sanitary and fills your expectations of what a

pleasant spa experience should be (most are not cheap). Talk to
the receptionist and find out how the spa differs from others.
Many spas offer food, tea, and coffee and cater to serving you
and making you feel pampered. Other spas may be more clinical.

It is best to book appointments at least a week in advance,
and multiple bookings may require a month or more of advance
booking. For optimal results, it is best to schedule massages
every four weeks. Be sure the massage therapists, estheticians,
nutritionists, and other staff members are licensed and well
trained. Many spas now have detailed Web sites, so these facts
should be listed.

The day spa offerings may vary, depending on the clientele
and location. For instance, one popular spa near one of our clinics offers the following different types of massage, which are
explained in the next step:

Detox Rejuvenating Full Body Skin Polish and Massage
Deep Massage
Effleurage Massage
Reflexology Massage
Upper Back, Neck, and Scalp Massage
Acupressure/Shiatsu Massage
Therapeutic Stress Body Massage
Swedish Massage
Lymphatique Body Treatment Massage

You can expect to pay fifty dollars or more for a thirty-minute
massage. However, according to many of my patients, this personal relaxation time is worth every penny and allows them to
stay active and get back to their regular routine.

CREATE YOUR OWN SPA EXPERIENCE

If you cannot afford a day spa experience or cannot find time to
visit one, create your own spa environment. Daily exercise is
essential for good health. Spending time in nature while gardening, biking on trails, walking in the woods, or swimming is

great for the body and soul. Don't forget to stretch before and after exercise and breathe in the fresh, outdoor air.

As you prepare for sleep, a soothing warm bath is a good idea to help the muscles relax. Surround your bathtub with glowing aromatic candles as you do your soothing moist heat soak. Add Dead Sea salts (available at department stores or online), Epsom salts, and/or aromatherapy essential oils to your liking. Play a favorite New Age or classical CD during your moist heat soak, and let the background music help eliminate negative thoughts as you focus on the calmness of the moment.

It's important to remember the feet and hands as you create your spa experience. With massage oil, cream, or lotion, take time to really moisturize and massage your hands and feet. If there are any sore or tender spots, focus on pressing on these areas and relieving the built-up stress. This is wonderful, especially if you are on your feet much of the day.

After your bath, do some relaxing stretches or gentle yoga positions (see pages 124 to 130), and focus on deep and full breathing to calm the mind and prepare for quality sleep. Before you turn back the covers, dab several drops of naturally sedating lavender oil on a clean handkerchief, and place it on your pillow for instant relief from the day's tensions. Invest in an eye pillow that you can place over your eyes to help relax tense eye and forehead muscles.

Balance Your Life to Reduce Stress

In short, I know coping with the ongoing stress of fibromyalgia is not easy, but it is an important step in the treatment plan. High levels of stress can add to the wear-and-tear levels on your body and contribute to the pain, fatigue, and depression you already feel. This, in turn, can make it even more difficult to handle other problems that confront you each day.

As you begin to reduce stress in your life, work for an overall lifestyle balance. Make time to do the things you *want* to do, as well as the things you *have* to do. People with chronic diseases are faced with special demands that healthy people do not have. The task of coping with pain and fatigue each day makes it necessary to keep your priorities in order so you have the energy to reach your daily goals.

Remember, no matter what type of disease, all people with pain are stressed. Likewise, all people with fatigue are stressed. When you combine these two major symptoms in a disease like fibromyalgia, it makes it even more difficult to handle everyday issues, much less major life stressors that may arise. Although only you can get your life in control, do not feel as if you must do this alone. There are trained professionals ready to guide you and your family in a positive direction that will help you to understand and accept your illness and learn to live a quality life—doing the things you want to do—without restraint.

7

STEP 4:
TRY A COMPLEMENTARY
APPROACH TO RELIEF

Because fibromyalgia has no single mode of treatment but depends on specific lifestyle changes, you may discover that a complementary approach to healing is very effective in soothing the symptoms of pain, depression, and fatigue.

My patients tell of using safe forms of alternative or complementary treatment along with their regular medical regime. This treatment may include chiropractic, massage, acupuncture, and herbal or dietary supplements. Some find that a combination of complementary treatments—along with the medications, moist heat, and exercise—add a boost for healing, especially for chronic muscle pain that is unending.

Because the efficacy of many popular complementary forms of treatment has hardly been proven, it is important to weigh the pros and cons of using each, and evaluate the benefit to the disease. In my three clinics, it is only after discussing this individually with each patient that I offer my support and only if the following two criteria are met:

1. If the patient finds that the complementary treatment makes her feel better
2. If the complementary treatment does not hurt the patient in any way

Let's look at some of the most common forms of complementary treatment.

Massage

When you are very stressed and your muscles are tense, they build up lactic acid. This makes the muscles even more tense. Massage, a holistic philosophy for pain management, may help to relieve this.

Studies released from the University of Miami School of Medicine's Touch Research Center found that the benefits of massage include heightened alertness, relief from depression and anxiety, an increase in the number of natural "killer cells" in the immune system, lower levels of the stress hormone cortisol, and reduced difficulty in getting to sleep.

Another study reported that patients who received massage for pain-related ailments took fewer narcotics or sedatives for the pain—an important benefit for FMS patients. The patients have reported a decreased heart rate and blood pressure and even a reduced skin temperature.

In an Internet survey published in the *Journal of the American Academy of Nurse Practitioners* (August 2000), sixty participants submitted an online questionnaire on fibromyalgia and alternative therapies. Massage was among the top interventions tried by patients and was ranked as one of the most effective complementary treatments. In another study reported in the *Archives of Internal Medicine,* massage was found to be therapeutic for persistent low-back pain.

Of course, massage affects the body as a whole. This form of drugless or alternative therapy has been shown to increase circulation, give relief from musculoskeletal pain, act as a mind/body form of stress relief, and increase flexibility and mobility. While massage therapy may seem to be "mechanical" in form, there is a great artistic component with various manual techniques—gliding, rubbing, kneading, tapping, cupping, manipulating, hacking, holding, friction pressure, and vibrating—using primarily the hands.

Many fibromyalgia patients find that massage gives relief of muscle pain and stiffness, even though it may be temporary relief, lasting hours or a few days. In one study, researchers gave twice-weekly massage for thirty minutes each session to a group of fibromyalgia patients. This study extended for five weeks. Afterward the investigators found that the participants who received massage increased the number of hours of sleep, and the number of tender points decreased, as did the levels of substance P.

Massage therapy also:

- relieves muscle spasm and tension.
- relieves tension-related headaches and headaches associated with FMS.
- strengthens the immune system.
- reduces blood pressure.
- improves digestion.
- creates a calmer mind/body state.
- relaxes nervous system and reduces anxiety.
- releases endorphins (natural painkillers).
- can increase the levels of serotonin (a natural antidepressant).

There are several popular massage techniques:

1. General Swedish is the foundation for all other types of massage with particular attention paid to the back and chest. It helps to flush the tissue of lactic and uric acids and other metabolic wastes, as well as to improve circulation in the body without increasing the load on the heart.

2. Trigger point is a type of massage and pain-relief technique that helps to alleviate muscle spasms and cramping. This type has been found helpful for many with FMS. The therapist will locate active and latent trigger points, and mild to moderate pressure is applied for a short time (about seven to ten seconds). The muscles are then gently stretched to help the relaxation process.

3. Deep Muscle Massage is applied with greater pressure and at deeper layers of the muscle than Swedish massage and is used to release chronic patterns of muscular tension using slow strokes, friction, or direct pressure. Often the movements are directed across the grain of the muscles (cross-fiber) using the fingers, thumbs, or elbows.

Other bodywork techniques may help deep-muscle pain, as well as other symptoms of fibromyalgia:

1. The Alexander Technique is a type of bodywork that is said to release painful muscle tension, improve posture, and reduce stress and fatigue.

2. Hellerwork is a therapy whereby the practitioner combines hands-on massage, movement, and dialogue to help you release accumulated stress and rigidity. Hellerwork is effective for temporary pain or tension relief.

3. Polarity therapy is a therapy where the practitioner uses gentle body manipulation and holding of pressure points to help restore natural energy flow. The practitioner will also educate you in exercise, nutrition, food combining, and maintaining a positive attitude to keep energy fields balanced.

4. Reiki is a type of bodywork based on the same energetic principles as tai chi and acupuncture. The Reiki healer rests her hands on various parts of your body in patterns that include the head, abdomen, legs, back, and feet. You may feel a sensation of warmth during this treatment.

5. Rolfing/Structural Integration is a therapy that promotes natural healing by realigning the body's underlying structure. The practitioner, or "rolfer," uses fingers, knuckles, and elbows to "sculpt" the client's body into correct alignment. This deep pressure applied by the rolfer helps to stretch the muscles and *fascia,* thick elastic connective tissue that envelops and supports muscles, tendons, and bones, making them more flexible.

6. Trager Method is a method of alternative healing that involves the use of movements, stretching, and pressure to help you give up muscular and mental tension and sink into a feeling of deep relaxation. Practitioners use movements such as gentle rocking, swinging, stretching, and pressure to help you get into a very deep state of relaxation.

7. Aston-Patterning is a method of muscle manipulation where the therapist uses a special "spiraling" technique to relax muscles and loosen tight joints. This method is said to help the body revert to a healthier posture. The Aston-Patterning therapist teaches clients how to keep muscle patterns healthy by changing environmental situations (the way you sit, stand, sleep).

8. Feldenkrais is a form of bodywork that teaches you to make body movement a conscious act. The therapist will educate you in how to sit, stand, and move, allowing your body to work with the force of gravity instead of against it, thus alleviating abnormal pressure and pain.

9. Myofascial Release is a way of stretching the body tissue to release tension in the fascia and make posture changes in alignment. The goal of the therapist is to gently elongate the tissue to help ease muscle pain.

10. Watsu (meaning water shiatsu) is a relatively new form of bodywork that takes place in chest-high warm water. With watsu, the therapist gives a gentle massage, working to stretch tightened muscles, and then engages clients in flowing, dance-like movements to alleviate tension and bottled-up emotions that can lead to muscle pain. The main benefit of watsu is that the water's buoyancy helps to relieve painful tissues and joints, while providing an ease of movement that is virtually impossible on land. During the session, you might float in the water horizontally so your spine is freed from gravitational strain. This

gives the benefit of alleviating tension and bottled-up emotions
that are tightening muscles and joints.

If you would like to find a qualified and licensed massage
therapist, the American Massage Therapy Association provides
a national referral service for qualified, professional massage
therapists (see Resources, page 286).

SELF-HELP FOR MUSCLE TENSION

Neck pain? Take two tennis balls and put them in a sock. Lie
down on a firm surface and put the balls behind your neck, just
beneath the shelf of the skull. Close your eyes and breathe deeply,
then gradually reposition the balls further down your neck.

Tense muscles? Lie on the floor or back up against a wall and
position the ball where you find intense soreness. The ball will
add pressure to painful trigger points, similar to the way acupressure or acupuncture works.

Chinese Medicine

Chinese medicine is another alternative treatment many are
turning to for fibromyalgia relief. This is a complete health system that has been used for more than five thousand years and is
comprised of exercises, herbal medicine, massage, nutrition,
and healthy living. Unlike Western medicine, which relies on
aggressive and invasive action of surgery or modern drugs. Chinese medicine tries to diagnose disturbances of *qi,* or *vital
energy,* in health and disease. Practitioners correct this dishar-
mony in the body using acupressure, acupuncture, shiatsu,
herbal medicine, Oriental massage, qigong, or tai chi.

According to proponents, traditional Chinese medicine has
therapeutic value in the treatment of chronic hepatitis, rheumatoid arthritis, headaches, fibromyalgia, menstrual cramps, lower
back and neck pain, substance abuse, hypertension, atopic
eczema, immunologic disorders, and acquired immunodeficiency
syndrome (AIDS). Although some scientific studies conclude

that acupuncture and some herbs may have medicinal value, most Chinese therapies still need to be studied in the United States using the highest research criteria.

Acupressure is a well-known ancient form of physical therapy that was discovered before *acupuncture,* using the same points. This type of Chinese medicine therapy works by stimulating your body's main "trigger points" to release energy or unblock qi. Today, acupressure is mainly used to help alleviate pain associated with sinus pressure, leg cramps, headaches, temporomandibular joint (TMJ) disorder, and carpal tunnel syndrome.

Acupuncture is a form of hyperstimulation for pain relief. There seems to be a close correlation between "tender points" and acupuncture sites used for pain control. A study published in the *British Medical Journal* (May 27, 1995) compared two groups of patients with fibromyalgia. One group was treated with electroacupuncture and the other was given sham treatment during which acupuncture needles were inserted but somewhat less deeply, at a small distance from usually prescribed acupuncture sites, and with a slightly weaker electric current. There was improvement in actively treated patients in terms of duration of morning stiffness, overall pain, sleep quality, and overall assessment of disease compared with baseline. There was no significant improvement in the control group. These results were comparable to those reported for some medical treatments such as with the antidepressant drug Elavil, or amitriptyline (see page 74).

There are new findings that acupuncture may be an excellent treatment for fibromyalgia symptoms. For instance, investigators from the University of Pennsylvania Medical Center used advanced imaging equipment to view the brains of nine patients—four pain sufferers and five healthy people—while they underwent acupuncture. Researchers said they saw blood flow increase in the thalamus, a kind of relay station for pain messages in the brain, along with other changes in the brain stem and cortex. In a recent study presented at the annual meeting of the American College of Rheumatology in November 2001, investigators concluded that acupuncture was a viable treatment for the pain and depression associated with fibromyalgia. Over a sixteen-week period, patients with fibromyalgia were evaluated for pain, depression, and quality of life. While all patients received amitriptyline, a commonly used pain modifier for fibromyalgia, twenty of the women received once-a-week acupuncture sessions for thirty minutes. The other group received "sham" sessions. Researchers reported that those women who received the real acupuncture sessions were the only ones who showed measurable improvement in pain, mental health, and depression after the first month.

In another study published in the journal *Wiener Klinische Wochenschrift* (July 2000), investigators treated tender points in fibromyalgia patients with acupuncture. Researchers found that the number of tender points was reduced and the temperature of the skin was reduced, suggesting that the circulation in the tender areas was also improved by the acupuncture treatments.

Western medicine research into the subject tells us that acupuncture brings relief through certain reflexes in the body that occur by way of the nervous system. That is to say by stimulating one portion of the body and using pathways of the nervous system, an effect is obtained in the same or another portion of the body. Additionally, it is believed that acupuncture causes the body to release endorphins that are the body's own pain-relieving chemicals.

Traditional Asian acupuncturists place the needles into specific acupuncture points along your body on lines known as meridians. Western doctors many times use the same points and may additionally use local trigger points, knotted areas in the muscle, which may be responsible for causing the localized or referred pain. Sometimes a slight electrical current is added (electroacupuncture). Acupuncture may therefore assist those with chronic, deep muscle pain, such as the case with fibromyalgia patients.

If you try acupuncture, with your doctor's approval, you need to go through a series of at least eight to ten treatments in order to ascertain whether it will be effective for you. You may not feel any relief, or you may feel extremely long-lasting relief. However, be sure that you go to a licensed practitioner who uses disposable needles.

Shiatsu is another form of Asian therapy where the therapist focuses on relieving pain and helping your body rid itself of any toxins before they develop into illness. Firm, rhythmic pressure is applied for three to ten seconds on specific points. The practitioner will try to awaken the meridians, or healing channels, of the body. Scientifically, this applied pressure may stimulate your body's *endorphins* to produce a tranquilizing effect, or it may help by loosening up muscles and improving blood circulation.

Shiatsu may have great benefit to those with FMS, as it is said to help ease or eliminate back pain and sciatica, digestive problems, headaches, insomnia, leg and menstrual cramps, respiratory problems, and shoulder stiffness.

Chiropractic

Does chiropractic really work? It all depends on what it is used for. Chiropractic medicine comes closer to traditional Western medicine than the other forms described in this chapter. It is a drug-free approach to health that relies on manipulation of the spine and muscles.

Doctors of chiropractic are unique in that instead of treating the symptoms of a patient, they are primarily interested in treating the spinal bones when they lose their normal position and motion from stress, trauma, or other causes.

According to doctors of chiropractic, your nervous system controls all functions in your body; every cell in your body is supplied with nervous impulses. Messages must travel from your brain down your spinal cord, then out to nerves to the particular parts of the body, and then back to the spinal cord and back up to the brain. The theory is that abnormal positions of the spinal bones may interfere with these messages and oftentimes are the underlying cause of many health problems.

Doctors of chiropractic correct the abnormal positions of the spinal bones with what is called an adjustment or spinal manipulation. The doctor's hands or a specially designed instrument deliver a brief and accurate thrust. This adjustment involves the use of a specific force in a precise direction applied to a joint that is fixated, locked up, or not moving properly. Adjustments help return the bones to a more normal position or motion, relieving pain and ill health.

The chiropractic doctor will also recommend a program of rehabilitation for your spine. This phase of care is analogous to orthodontics. Goals are to stabilize and reduce joint involvement, rehabilitate muscle ligament tissue, and balance nerve impulses, helping you to regain maximum health.

Chiropractic care for some types of chronic pain is not without scientific substantiation. In a new report published in the *Annals of Internal Medicine* (May 2002), researchers compared three different treatments for neck pain in 183 patients with chronic neck pain. The groups received either routine medical care by a physician (pain medications and rest), physical therapy (active exercises), or manual therapy (manual manipulation of the neck).

After seven weeks of treatment, the manual therapy group had the best outcome with 68.3 percent of the patients saying the therapy had helped ease the pain. About half or 50.8 percent of the patients who had physical therapy reported relief, and only 35.9 percent of the patients who were under a physician's medical care felt relief. Patients who do get significant relief from spinal manipulation find that it helps them to continue with their basic treatment plan of moist heat and exercises and allows them to resume a normal lifestyle. Additionally, manipulation by a doctor of chiropractic, osteopathy, or other practitioner can be part of a total team approach to treatment with a neurologist, orthopedic surgeon, or rheumatologist to bring about the best total results for that patient.

Biofeedback

Biofeedback is based on the idea that when people are given information about their body's internal processes, they can use this information to learn to control those processes. This type of therapy has been shown to bring about improvement in the number of tender points, visual analogue pain, and morning stiffness in some fibromyalgia patients. In a study demonstrating the impact of biofeedback on FMS patients, fifteen patients who had a poor response to medication treatment were trained with biofeedback. After a fifteen-session electromyographic (EMG) biofeedback program, these patients improved in tender point count, pain rating, and morning stiffness.

Biofeedback requires you to be connected to a machine that informs you and your therapist when you are physically relaxing your body. With sensors placed over specific muscle sites, the therapist will read the tension in your muscles, the amount of sweat produced, or the measurement of finger temperature. Any one or all of these readings can let the trained biofeedback therapist know if you are learning to relax. When taught by a qualified licensed psychologist, with biofeedback the patient can control responses of the body, resulting in control of pain and stress.

The ultimate goal of biofeedback is to use this skill outside the therapist's office when you are facing real stressors. If learned successfully, electronic biofeedback can help you control your heart rate, blood pressure, and muscle tension when you are not hooked up to the machine. Some therapists recommend relaxation tapes that can be listened to at home to practice relaxation techniques.

Biofeedback has been found helpful in relieving temporomandibular joint (TMJ) dysfunction, neck and shoulder pain, anxiety, irritable bowel syndrome (IBS), epilepsy, asthma, Raynaud's syndrome, hypertension, and incontinence. Some common types of biofeedback include:

Electromyographic (EMG) biofeedback. This type provides feedback on muscle tension and works well for patients with anxiety disorders or chronic pain.

Electrodermal (EDR) biofeedback. This type of biofeedback measures subtle changes in amounts of perspiration.

Thermal biofeedback. The temperature of the skin is measured and is used in teaching hand warming. This has been found to help relieve migraine headaches and can benefit those with Raynaud's disease.

Finger pulse biofeedback. The finger pulse records heart rate and force and is useful for anxiety or cardiovascular symptoms.

Respiration feedback. This type of biofeedback shows the rate, volume, rhythm, and location of each breath.

Hydrotherapy

Hydrotherapy works by stimulating your body's own healing force. Cold compresses reduce swelling by constricting blood vessels that help to control minor internal bleeding. Moist heating pads, whirlpools, or even a warm shower can reduce the soreness of aching or inflamed muscles. Even the simple act of running cool water over a wound can help rid it of dangerous bacteria and aid in healing.

The most common forms of hydrotherapy—ice and moist heat—are right at your fingertips. The next time you have unyielding muscle pain, use moist heat—a warm shower, a moist heating pad, a whirlpool spa, or even warm water running over the injury, sore muscle, or aching arthritic joint. For a new injury, apply the R.I.C.E. theory—Rest, Ice, Compression, and Elevation.

Detoxification

Detoxification is centuries old, going back to early biblical times when fasting was used as a method of spiritual cleansing. Avoidance of chemicals, from food or other sources, refined food, sugar, caffeine, alcohol, tobacco, and drugs is a safe way to detoxify your body and helps to minimize the toxic load.

Detoxification on a simple level makes practical sense, if you follow a healthful cleansing routine of exercise and sweat, fresh fruits and vegetables, increased liquids with more frequent urination, or more sleep when under stress. Yet the age-old theories behind colon cleansing or lengthy fasts are just that—ancient theories. In fact, many cleansing plans should not be done by expectant mothers, diabetics, and those who have chronic illnesses such as heart, kidney, or lung disease. Until research promotes these methods as safe and effective with substantial scientific evidence, stick to detox methods that you know to be safe.

Hypnotherapy

Hypnosis is another way to control the pain and stress that accompany fibromyalgia and has been highly endorsed by the American Psychiatric Association and the American Psychological Association. Although the word *hypnosis* comes from the Greek meaning "sleep," it is really an intense state of focused concentration.

In one controlled trial, hypnotherapy patients reported a better outcome with respect to their pain experience, fatigue on awakening, and sleep pattern as compared to patients receiving physical therapy.

Although this is not a "new" method of treatment, it is now being used in newer ways to improve the quality of life of chronic-pain patients. With hypnosis, suggestions are made to the patient during a session that allow her to decrease the intensity of the pain, to move the pain to another area, or to try to build a feeling of separation from the pain.

Although this may sound too easy to work, hypnosis has been used successfully to help chronic pain in limited studies. I recommend that it be used to supplement other methods of pain control (such as exercises and medications).

If done correctly, this type of mind-body therapy can ideally produce a feeling of calm and improve a patient's confidence in handling the symptoms of fibromyalgia. Because hypnosis is not meant for everyone and may not work in every person, you should seek a qualified clinical psychologist or psychiatrist to help you decide if hypnosis would be helpful and safe for you.

Environmental Medicine

It makes sense that what we eat, breathe, wear, or sleep on can ultimately affect how we think, feel, act, and react. According to environmental medicine proponents, a wide range of toxic or harmful substances, including foods and chemicals found in the air, water, and food, can cause illness in the body. These environmental toxins, including processed foods and food additives, can tear down the body, resulting in poor emotional and psychological health.

Depending on your locale, exposure to toxins may affect your nervous system, lungs, and even your immune function. In some cases, it may have a bearing on your FMS. In fact, research studies support the use of environmental medicine for allergies, arthritis, asthma, chemical sensitivity, colitis, depression, panic attacks, reduced attention spans, eczema, fatigue, and hyperactivity. The treatment focuses on eliminating the environmental hazardous sources we can control. You may be told to modify your diet and to avoid such deleterious substances as strong shampoos, aerosol deodorants, cigarette smoke, exhaust fumes, organic solvents and pesticides, plastics, paints, perfumes and colognes, medications, gas used for cooking and heating, building materials, synthetic fibers, and certain clothing.

To see if the theory behind environmental medicine may help alleviate your symptoms, go through your home or office, and discover the problem areas. While environmental triggers vary, common triggers include aerosols, chemical fumes, cockroaches, cold air, dust, fresh paint, humid air, mold and mildew, perfume and scented products, pet dander, pollen, tobacco smoke, and wood smoke.

Removing those toxins you can control, and focusing on natural foods and household cleaning products, may help you to think clearer, avoid fibro fog, and even regulate your moods.

Light Therapy

Light therapy is an up-and-coming alternative treatment that involves using natural or artificial light to cause physiological changes in the human body. Most recently, doctors are using light therapy to relieve the symptoms associated with seasonal affective disorder (SAD), a psychological problem that occurs with the change of seasons and less sunlight exposure. Those who have SAD feel depressed and fatigued, and may crave carbohydrates, as these carbohydrates boost levels of serotonin in the body.

Using specially made "light boxes," people are exposed to bright light and their bodies subsequently produce serotonin. In comprehensive studies on light therapy, women participants with PMS reported less depression, less moodiness, better sleep, and better concentration. Researchers have shown that serotonin levels drop just before ovulation, and this drop correlates with the onset of PMS symptoms; serotonin levels rebound with the onset of menstruation or when PMS symptoms decrease. Recent research suggests that PMS occurs in women with low base levels of serotonin; when serotonin levels drop further at ovulation, these levels fall low enough for symptoms to appear. Using phototherapy, women with PMS can keep their serotonin-melatonin levels high enough to prevent their PMS symptoms from appearing.

Because of the boost of serotonin, light therapy may ease the depression associated with fibromyalgia. In fact, many mildly depressed individuals have seen improvement with just thirty minutes of bright light exposure; others may need up to two hours daily. This is consistent with the belief that light therapy helps people with winter depression because it makes up for light lost during shorter winter days.

Aromatherapy

This type of complementary "nose-mind" therapy involves the ancient art of using fragrances or essential and absolute oils and other substances for physical and psychological benefits. *Essential oil* is an extract or essence that's been distilled, usually by steam, from the seed, leaves, stem, flower, bark, root, or other parts of a plant, and an *absolute oil* is a very concentrated liquid taken from a plant and is extracted by alcohol. Essential oils are often diluted in a *carrier oil* such as sweet almond, grapeseed, olive, or canola oil before using with massage.

Each of the different aromas or oils has a specific healing power, whether to reduce stress, fight infection, increase productivity, or serve as an aphrodisiac. For example, lavender and spiced apples are said to increase the alpha-wave activity in the back of the brain, which leads to relaxation. Increased beta activity in the front of the brain, on the other hand, shows greater alertness and is said to occur with the smell of jasmine or lemon. Some research has found chamomile essential oil to be an anti-inflammatory, and clove oil is antimicrobial.

Although it has been found that odors can change brain-wave states, how do scientists explain this connection between odors and moods? Exactly how the scent-mood link works remains a mystery. Researchers do know that when aromatic molecules drift into the nose, they lock on to receptors there and create electrical impulses that travel up the olfactory nerves to the brain. One destination is the limbic system, where emotions and memory are processed. There is widespread agreement that these aromas help to increase the quality of sensory input for patients, thus reducing levels of stress.

Although there have been no controlled studies to date, claims rest on patients who say to have been healed or at least made to feel better with aromatherapy. Therefore, the answer as to whether scents can change one's mood and reduce stress could actually lie with each person. Sometimes fragrant oils are used in conjunction with therapeutic touch to ease the tension on the skin surface. These oils not only feel soothing to the touch, but also have scents that can evoke tranquillity.

There are two national professional organizations, the National Association for Holistic Aromatherapy and the American Alliance of Aromatherapy, along with a host of treatment centers across the nation specializing in this mind/body approach to healing and pain relief.

To use essential oils, try the following:

- Inhale the oil by adding 5 to 10 drops to steaming water or to a humidifier.
- Mix 1 teaspoon oil with 1 pint carrier oil, and use as a massage oil.
- Add 5 to 10 drops to warm bath water.
- Mix 5 drops with 1 cup warm water and mist into the air.
- Put 1 to 2 drops on top of the candle's melted wax, and inhale the warm scent.

ESSENTIAL OILS THAT RELIEVE STRESS

ESSENTIAL OIL	EFFECT ON THE BODY
Basil, rosemary, and lemon oil	Increases mental alertness
Lavender and chamomile	Relieves insomnia, PMS, and cramps
Sandalwood and geranium	Improves sex drive
Frankincense and marjoram	Soothes raw nerves
Jasmine and rose	Increases confidence
Lavender, vanilla, and chamomile	De-stresses

ESSENTIAL OIL	EFFECT ON THE BODY
Basil, geranium, and orange oil	Combats depression
Peppermint and geranium	Boosts creativity
Orange, peppermint, and rosemary	Increases energy
Sandalwood and peppermint	Soothes upset stomach

Mind-Body Therapies

As you've experienced, the daily stress of worrying about fibromyalgia and the limitations that accompany it can often put you in a state of emotional and mental overload.

The relaxation response, first described by Dr. Herbert Benson more than twenty years ago, is one of the most studied methods to reduce stress. Learning to induce the relaxation response at will can offer a real potential to reduce physical strain and emotional, negative thoughts—and increase your ability to self-manage stress.

Relaxation may be easy for some, but most people, even when they think they are relaxing, are not aware of the enormous muscle tension running throughout the body. However, by allowing time in your daily schedule to practice the suggested mind-body therapy and alternative treatment in this chapter, you can begin to get in touch with this muscle tension and learn how to end it—permanently.

Autogenics

Because the brain needs only a few reminders to calm down, autogenics teaches you to concentrate on raising the temperature of your hands and feet. Proponents claim that autogenics will give your heart a break from pumping so hard, open blood vessels, reduce breathing rate and pulse, and even lower blood pressure.

To do this relaxation technique, sit quietly, and put your left hand in your lap, palm up. Lay your right palm on top of your left palm, and clasp your fingers together. Concentrating on the feeling in your hands, *mindfully* (focus all attention on what you feel from moment to moment) work to raise the temperature of your hands for ten minutes. Then do the same with your feet. Counselors claim that if this is done correctly, you will feel "the heat" rise in both your hands and feet, indicating that your body is relaxing.

Laughter Therapy

Can a laugh a day keep FMS symptoms away? Maybe, according to many researchers. Laughter increases the activity of body cells that attack tumor cells and viruses. It helps to relieve anxiety, decreases stress-producing hormones, and increases immune system activity. In fact, many doctors are now prescribing "humor therapy" for chronically ill patients.

Norman Cousins was the first to promote laugher as an antidote to disease. While editor of the *Saturday Review,* Cousins was diagnosed with a serious connective tissue disease. After his doctors said that it was incurable, he was determined to get well.

During his journey to find a cure for his ailment, Cousins discovered that laughter actually affected his body chemistry in a positive, healing way. He filled his life with movies that made him laugh—"a real belly laugh." He then documented his account of the "miraculous recovery from laughter" in the book *Anatomy of an Illness as Perceived by the Patient.* As he recovered from his so-called incurable illness, Cousins went on to tell others of the miraculous power of laughter and about the resulting positive chemical changes in the body.

Today's scientists have found that laughing can produce a state of positive stress, or what is called *eustress.* In a study on laughter's effect on the immune system, researchers at Loma Linda University in California showed a video of a comedian.

Blood samples drawn during and after the video showed significant increases in various measures of immune function, particularly T cells and NK (natural killer) cells. Interestingly, the levels of the stress hormone cortisol, which suppress the immune system, were lower. The researchers concluded that laughter creates its own physiological state with positive changes in the immune system opposite those of negative stress or distress.

Meditation

Remember when transcendental meditation was thought to be a cult? Today meditation is recognized as a viable way to lower blood pressure, alleviate insomnia, and reduce chronic pain. This stress releaser seeks to integrate the mind, body, and spirit through intentionally focusing on the silent repetition of a focus word ("love"), sound ("om"), phrase ("peace heals"), or prayer ("thank you, God"). As thoughts intrude, you will continue to *mindfully* chant while facilitating the relaxation response.

This technique can guide you beyond the negative thoughts and agitations of the busy mind and allow you to become "unstuck" from your fear and other disturbing emotions.

Music Therapy

Music therapy has been proven to be an effective nonpharmacologic approach to assist in reducing fear, anxiety, stress, or grief in chronically ill patients. It is just beginning to make its mark as a way to treat pain and the stress that accompanies it, yet many are already reporting it as the best way to lower stress. Some researchers have found that in studies with chronic pain patients, the use of music can cause most patients to have a higher tolerance for pain.

Music therapy may sound too easy to work, but many of the sensations arising from music and pain are processed in the same areas of the brain. These areas are also responsible for coordinating our emotional responses. So, by focusing on and responding to music, perhaps we can block our bodies' response to pain. With this relaxation, we can decrease muscle tension and increase blood levels of endorphins. Although the level of pain does not change, having less tension and anxiety can make it tolerable.

For de-stressing, it is helpful to try music therapy in combination with another mind/body technique, such as deep abdominal breathing, progressive muscle relaxation, or guided imagery (visualization), as discussed in the following sections of this chapter.

If you employ music therapy as part of your treatment program, make sure that the pace of the music you choose is slightly slower than your heart rate, or approximately sixty beats a minute. This rhythm encourages your heart rate to slow down, and some studies of late have shown that this will also lower blood pressure. The works of Vivaldi and Chopin would fit this category, or you might try New Age music by artists such as George Winston with Windham Hill.

Deep Abdominal Breathing

Breathing can measure and alter your psychological state, making a stressful moment accelerate or diminish in intensity. Think about how your respiration quickens when you are fearful or in great pain, and how taking a deep, slow breath can have a calming effect, reducing both stress and levels of muscle pain.

Although we often take breathing for granted, this is one of the few activities of the body that we can consciously control. As you learn how to do deep abdominal breathing, you will gain control over a basic physiological function, helping to decrease the release of stress hormones and slow down your heart rate during stressful moments. Also, by adding oxygen to the blood, you can actually cause your body to release endorphins, the hormones that give a greater sense of well-being and contentment.

Lie on your back in a quiet room with no distractions. If necessary, take the phone off the hook so you are truly alone. Place your hands on your abdomen and take a slow, deliberate deep breath in through your nostrils. If your hands are rising, your abdomen is expanding and you are breathing correctly. If your hands do not rise, yet you see your chest rising, you are breathing incorrectly.

Inhale to a count of five, pause for three seconds, then exhale to a count of five. Start with ten repetitions of this exercise, and then increase to twenty-five, twice daily. Use this exercise any time you feel anxious or stressed. Some of my patients find it extremely helpful when they are experiencing great pain. As one patient, Laura, said, "When I have severe muscle pain, I use my breathing to go with the pain. Somehow, this takes my mind off the pain and lessens its severity."

Progressive Muscle Relaxation

Progressive muscle relaxation involves contracting and then relaxing all the different muscle groups in the body, beginning with head and neck and progressing down to the arms, chest, back, stomach, pelvis, legs, and feet. To do this exercise, you focus on each set of muscles, tense these muscles to the count of ten, and then release to the count of ten. Go slowly as you progress throughout your entire body, taking as long as you can. Get in touch with each part and feel the tension you are experiencing. Also, notice how it feels to be tension-free as you release the muscle.

Studies show that when you can create a strong mental image using this type of relaxation technique, you actually feel "removed" from cumbersome stress and negative emotions. This *mindfulness*, or focusing of attention, can also help you move beyond destructive habits as you become centered in a world of health and inner healing.

You can do this exercise with or without music, and it is important to perform it with deep abdominal breathing, focusing on your breath. Breathe in while tensing the muscles, and breathe out or exhale while relaxing them.

Guided Imagery Techniques

According to scientific tests, the mind cannot distinguish between fears, fantasies, and reality. Therefore, another effective mind-body technique for healing is guided imagery (also called visualization). This involves mentally seeing pictures of relaxing situations, such as a beach at sunset, a flowing mountain waterfall, or a brilliant mountain sunrise.

The power of your imagination is important in guided imagery, as you use sights, sounds, feelings, and smell to create a desired state in your mind. Used in combination with deep breathing, it produces long-term stress reduction. This technique has been used to improve the surveillance function of the immune system. Through guided imagery, you will reduce your anxiety level during stressful times and lower your heart rate and blood pressure. As you continuously visualize a positive healing image, you may significantly contribute to your own well-being.

If you have trouble imagining scenes and images, listen to sounds of waves or thunderstorms to trigger natural settings. Tapes can be purchased at any music store. Or, purchase postcards with peaceful, serene scenes on them, and keep these with you. Pull out your visualization cards when you feel your body tensing and you need to imagine being somewhere else where life is kinder and less threatening.

Prayer and Spirituality

Many fibromyalgia patients find great comfort in prayer as they allow their thoughts to take a break from daily analytical routines. During prayer or meditation, the body switches from the pumping "fight or flight" response into a calmer, more peaceful mood. Like other forms of mental aerobics, both prayer and meditation have been shown to produce alpha and theta waves consistent with happiness and serenity.

In findings presented at the Association of Rheumatology Health Professionals annual meeting (2001), investigators from the Johns Hopkins School of Medicine theorized that spirituality, meaning an inner intangible force that allows you to cope with life's challenges, is another psychological resource that can help people adjust to living with a chronic illness. In the study of patients with arthritis, researchers found that those patients who were spiritual were also more positive in their daily lives, had better coping skills than those who did not claim to be spiritual, and found meaning in their existence—even with a serious illness. It is thought that having a spiritual practice helps link us to others, through experiences, gatherings, personal outreach, and social support, providing a vital buffer against stress and emotional problems.

Homeopathic Medicine

Homeopathic remedies are regulated by the Food and Drug Administration (FDA). Proponents believe that this form of alternative medicine effectively treats allergic rhinitis, hay fever, migraine headaches, trauma, gastritis, allergic asthma, acute childhood diarrhea, fibromyalgia, and influenza. Yet lack of convincing scientific proof is one of the great problems with homeopathy's acceptance by conventional medical doctors. Critics believe that because the medications are so diluted, the only benefit received is placebo.

Nonetheless, a survey of 107 clinical trials published in the *British Medical Journal* (February 1991) showed that 80 percent were positive in favor of homeopathy. One landmark review published in the scientific journal *The Lancet* said that homeopathy was shown to be nearly two and a half times more effective than placebos in the treatment of such problems as arthritis, allergies, varicose veins, and gastrointestinal pain.

Some commonly used homeopathic remedies include:

Aconitum for PMS
Allium cepa for allergies and colds
Arnica for sore muscles, bruises, and sprains
Belladonna for PMS and menopausal symptoms
Bryonia for constipation and vaginal dryness
Chamomilla for earache and PMS
Cimicifuga for PMS, anxiety, and depression
Cocculus for depression and sleep deprivation
Colocynthis for menstrual cramps and irritability
Conium maculatum for breast tenderness and swelling
Gelsemium for headache
Ignatia amara for depression and sadness
Lachesis for PMS, headaches, pain, menopausal symptoms
Natrum muriatcum for menopausal symptoms
Nux vomica for diarrhea, hemorrhoids, and constipation
Sepia for PMS, menopausal symptoms, and depression

If you seek advice from a homeopathic practitioner, be sure this person is a medical doctor. Ask where he or she has studied homeopathy and whether a certification exam was passed. Licensing is required in only three states at this time, and there are no formal guidelines or formal schools for homeopathy. It is also imperative that you check with your own physician before taking any unknown substance or supplement because of the possibility of allergic reactions.

Herbal Therapy

Herbal and other plant-derived remedies have been estimated by the World Health Organization (WHO) to be the most frequently used therapies worldwide. Although precise levels of use in the United States are unknown, in 1994 herbal products accounted for sales of more than $1.6 billion, the fastest-growing category in drugstores.

Pharmaceutical companies are very interested in herbal therapy, and reports show that more than 25 percent of all prescription drugs are derived from these wild medicinals, including the flowers, leaves, bark, berries, and roots of plants. Although there are a few herbs that are dangerous and should never be ingested or put on your skin, most herbs are safe.

Keep in mind that if you do choose an herbal therapy, some therapeutic agents derived from plants include pure chemical entities available as prescription drugs (e.g., morphine). Plant-derived remedies can contain chemicals with potent pharmaco-logic toxicologic properties.

The problem with trying to purchase herbs that are "guaran-teed safe" is that there is no proof that herbal therapies work other than word of mouth from consumers. The reason for this is that in order to get FDA approval, the company marketing the drug must prove that it is safe and effective. Plants cannot be patented, so most companies call herbs "foods" and market them in this way.

Herbal remedies have been used for generations and can be put in tea or soup or taken in other forms. Certain remedies such as alfalfa or chamomile are more popular in some areas of this country than in others. Although some herbal therapies have not been shown to have a specific benefit for arthritis symptoms, some patients have used the following with good results for help-ing to obtain more restful sleep or for more energy.

HERBAL TREATMENTS

NAME OF HERB	COMMON USES
Astragalus	Stimulates immune function and triggers the production of interferon in fighting disease.
Blackcurrant seed oil	Suppresses inflammation and joint tissue injury.
Boswellia	Relieves inflammation.
Cayenne	Acts as a pain reliever. Relieves migraine or tension headaches.

	As a salve or ointment, relieves muscle pain.
Chamomile	Helps calm nervousness, anxiety, menstrual cramps, and upset stomach. May boost immune function.
Devil's Claw	Acts as an anti-inflammatory in the body and is used to treat migraines, back pain, and menstrual cramps.
Echinacea	Boosts the immune system and helps to prevent infections.
Feverfew	Inhibits inflammation and acts similarly to aspirin.
Ginger	Stimulates mucus-producing vagus nerve reflexes and has an antioxidant effect and an anti-inflammatory effect.
Ginkgo biloba	Improves concentration and memory, increases blood flow, and helps the symptoms of PMS. Helps with short-term memory loss and depression.
Ginseng	Increases energy and relieves stress.
Goldenseal	Soothes inflammation of the respiratory, digestive, and genitourinary tracts caused by allergy or infection.
Goto kola	As "brain food," promotes memory, alleviates mental fatigue, and normalizes blood pressure. Helps to improve mental ability and relieves stress.
Hawthorn berries	Strengthens the muscles and nerves to the heart.

NAME OF HERB	COMMON USES
Hyssop	Regulates blood pressure and promotes circulation. Relieves hoarseness, lung congestion, and mucus buildup.
Kava kava	Helps to fend off anxiety and nervous tension. Also has anti-inflammatory effect on the body.
Kelp	Provides energy and endurance, helps to relieve nervous tension, and promotes circulation to the brain.
Lavender	Relieves insomnia, depression, and headache.
Licorice	Promotes healthy adrenal glands and acts as a sexual stimulant.
Meadowsweet	Acts to reduce inflammation.
Milk thistle	Bolsters the immune system.
Myrrh	Cleans the colon and soothes digestive system upset.
Nettle	Contains a variety of natural chemicals that may help to lower pain, reduce swelling, and ease inflammation. These chemicals help slow down the actions of many enzymes that trigger inflammation.
Passionflower	Acts as a mild tranquilizer and eases insomnia, stress, and anxiety.
Pine bark	Stimulates circulation and helps reduce inflammation.
Psyllium	Helps to restore tone to the intestines and lubricates and heals irritated tissues.
Pycnogenol	Boosts serotonin in the body.
Saint-John's-wort	Relieves depression without the side effects of prescription antidepressants.

Slippery elm	Relieves sore throats and soothes mucous membranes.
Turmeric	Acts as a power anti-inflammatory and has a potent compound, curcumin, that protects the body against the ravages of free radicals, naturally occurring toxic substances.
Valerian	Acts as a sedative and helps to combat insomnia.
White willow bark	Decreases inflammation and acts as an "aspirin" substitute.

TAKE A CAUTIOUS APPROACH TO HERBAL THERAPY

If you want to try herbal therapy, it is important to consult with your physician. Many times you may pick up something at the grocery or health food store because of an advertised "quick cure" for pain and stiffness, but when it comes to self-medicating with herbs, my advice is usually "let the buyer beware." Always know what you are putting in your body and on your skin. When herbal therapies are not approved by the FDA, they can be combined with other ingredients that could actually make your condition worse. In other words, while most might help your symptoms, others can be deadly.

Some patients have taken products containing ephedra, thinking it might help boost alertness and energy. It's important to know that the FDA recently proposed cracking down on the marketing of ephedra products, citing about eight hundred injuries and at least seventeen deaths linked to the herbal stimulant. Among the proposals are limiting concentrations of the herb in any dietary supplement, requiring warning labels that its use can cause death, and banning claims that it can help people lose weight or build muscle. Some popular products containing ephedrine include "Herbal Ecstasy," "Ultimate Xphoria," and "Herbal Phen-Fen." It is also marketed as ma huang, Chinese ephedra, and epitonin.

Watch Herb-Drug Interactions

Just because an herb is "natural" does not mean it's always safe. If you are taking any medication, check with your doctor before self-medicating with herbal therapies. While herb-drug interactions are rare, they do occur. Because of possible dangerous interactions, do not use herbal therapies if you are taking any of the following medications: cyclosporine, digoxin, hypoglycemic agents, lithium, phenytoin, procainamide, theophylline, tricyclic antidepressants, and warfarin.

Natural Dietary Supplements

Dietary supplements include a host of products that contain vitamins, minerals, herbs, and amino acids as well as natural enzymes, organ tissues, metabolites, extracts, or concentrates. Some alternative practitioners recommend the following natural remedies for prevention and treatment of disease. Most are available at drugstores, grocery stores, or health food stores.

Chromium picolate is a trace mineral important in helping cells break down sugar into energy for the body. Supplements can help to regulate blood sugar, fat, and carbohydrate metabolism. Uncontrolled blood sugar levels can contribute to weight gain, high cholesterol, and high blood pressure. Interestingly, chromium seems to normalize low blood sugar. A recent USDA study of 180 Type 2 diabetics in China documented "spectacular" results from taking 1,000 micrograms of chromium picolinate daily with nearly all of the subjects no longer having the classic signs of diabetes. For those with FMS, taking chromium may help in stabilizing mood swings and anxiety caused by fluctuations in blood sugar levels.

CLA (conjugated linoleic acid) is a fatty acid that is said to reduce fat by inhibiting the body's ability to store fats. It also has antioxidant properties, increases muscle tone, and improves food efficiency.

Coenzyme Q10 is a natural substance that improves heart and immune function. It is also an antioxidant that helps to lower cholesterol levels and reduces oxidative damage to blood vessels.

Essential fatty acids (EFAs) are not manufactured by the body, but these fats are essential to cardiovascular health and normal brain development. EFAs are available in oils containing omega-3 (fish oils) and omega-6 (linolenic and gamma-linolenic, or GLA, which are found in plant oils such as evening primrose, black currant, and borage).

Glucosamine and **chondroitin** are two substances that the human body produces to make cartilage. In supplement form, glucosamine comes from crab shells, and chondroitin comes from cow cartilage. Although scientific studies have yet to call these the "cure" for arthritis, in some studies of people with arthritis, the supplements were found to ease aches as well as over-the-counter painkillers, but more slowly. Although their long-term safety has never been established, they appear to have no side effects, and researchers do not know whether you must take the two supplements together or if one is effective taken by itself. If you have osteoarthritis along with fibromyalgia, this natural solution may help you.

Lecithin is commercially isolated from soybeans, corn, and eggs and may help with easing the memory glitches that happen with aging. Just two tablespoons of lecithin a day stimulates the body's output of choline, a brain chemical that is important in recall and memory.

Get the Best of Both Worlds

It is important to be open-minded as you consider alternative treatments for fibromyalgia. You don't want to miss a chance for good relief, but you also don't want to take unnecessary risks.

When patients come to me with a new remedy that is an alternative treatment, I ask them to consider the following:

- Is it approved by the U.S. Food and Drug Administration (FDA)?
- Does it have any known side effects?
- What is the expertise of the person administering the remedy?
- What has happened to similar treatments over the years?
- Will your health insurance company reimburse you?

Become your own expert. Beware of any treatment that promises quick and easy relief or a cure. If it sounds too good to be true, it probably is! You can receive more information on alternative treatments from the Arthritis Foundation and the Fibromyalgia Association (see Resources, page 287).

It is important to know when a substance may be dangerous to your health, and you should avoid any substance taken internally. For example, rattlesnake meat is a common remedy in some areas for many illnesses, including arthritis and back pain. But some forms of capsules containing rattlesnake meat have been shown to cause serious illness.

If an alternative treatment is proven harmless and won't delay proper medical evaluation and treatment, then it is acceptable to try. If you have questions about a new treatment, talk to your doctor and make sure it is safe to use. This can allow you to take advantage of newer treatments, but avoid those that may cause more harm than relief.

It is my experience that once patients have the diagnosis of fibromyalgia and learn to live with it, they become the "experts" on their disease. Those who tell of feeling more energy and less pain have learned how to make lifestyle changes and use alternative and medical treatments in a complementary manner—in a way that enhances both health and well-being.

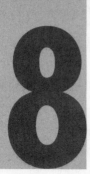

STEP 5:
END SLEEPLESS NIGHTS

Sleep deprivation was written all across Christina's face. Until she started treatment for fibromyalgia two years ago, this forty-seven-year-old woman lived for months with dark circles under her eyes from lack of restful sleep. Christina made it a point to be in bed by nine o'clock each night but then tossed and turned until sunrise and always felt too tired to go to work the next day.

Like Christina, the majority of fibromyalgia patients are fatigued, even after sleeping for ten hours at night. One woman said, "I go to bed tired and feel tired all night. I awaken tired, then I feel tired the next day."

Patients complain that no matter how long they sleep, it is never restful. Their sleep may be interrupted by frequent awakening, that is, becoming awake enough that they remember these times the next day. Even more common are awakenings that are not enough to remember but that definitely break up their deep sleep. Most patients tell of waking up day after day feeling exhausted. They feel more tired in the morning, and many have great difficulty in concentrating during the day, just as in other situations where sleep is disrupted.

Because obtaining restful sleep is a crucial problem with this disease, it is helpful to understand the characteristics of normal sleep and how this differs from the sleep experienced by fibro-myalgia patients.

Understanding the Stages of Sleep

Studies have demonstrated that we have a built-in cycle of sleep-wake times along with many other cyclic variations in bodily functions, such as glandular secretions, body tempera-ture, heart rate, blood pressure, and bronchial function. These intrinsic cycles are controlled by a group of nerve cells called a *circadian pacemaker.* This pacemaker is closely related to parts of the retina (in the back of the eye) and the hypothalamus in the brain.

The circadian cycle is actually twenty-five hours long. Since the cycle is longer than the twenty-four-hour day, some factor must serve to synchronize the body's pacemaker with the exter-nal clock time. These are cues from the environment called *zeit-gebers* (from German, meaning "time-givers"). The most important and powerful one is light. The hormone most closely linked to the circadian system is melatonin, which is made by the pineal gland in another part of the brain. Melatonin has been shown to synchronize the sleep-wake cycle to twenty-four hours in some blind subjects who were otherwise unable to live on a twenty-four-hour day.

In adults, sleep is made up of distinct types or stages with specific characteristics defined by brain waves, eye movements, and muscle tension. The two broad categories of sleep include rapid eye movement sleep (REM) and nonrapid eye movement sleep (NREM). During REM sleep, there are small, variable-speed brain waves, rapid eye movements like those of eyes-open wakefulness, and absent muscle tension. It is during REM sleep that we have almost all of our dreams. (Arousals from this stage of sleep are usually associated with recall of vivid imagery.) In NREM sleep, there are four different stages—1, 2, 3, and 4—characterized by different combinations of brain waves, eye movements, and reduced but not absent muscle tension. In fibromyalgia, stages 3 and 4 NREM sleep are of most importance. These stages are defined by relatively large, slow brain waves (delta waves), absent eye movements, and reduced muscle tension. Other names for these stages are "slow-wave sleep" or "delta sleep."

About sixty years ago, it was recognized that sleep intensity is reflected by the amount of delta sleep. The depth of sleep is correlated with this stage, and it is from delta sleep that arousal is most difficult. Interestingly, growth hormone secretion is highest during delta sleep. Some researchers suggest this is important for growth and repair of body tissue.

The stages of sleep can be contrasted with the state of wakefulness. The wake state is associated with small, variable, but mostly rapid (seven to eleven cycles per second) brain waves called *alpha waves*. There are quick, alert eye movements along with variable, generally high tension in the muscles.

The stages of sleep are distributed through the normal sleep period in a particular pattern. Sleep onset usually is within five to twenty minutes of going to bed. After the start of sleep, there is a cycling through stages 1 to 4 approximately every forty-five to ninety minutes with REM sleep punctuating each cycle at about sixty- to ninety-minute intervals. Delta sleep occurs mostly in the first third of the night and makes up about 10 to 20 percent of total nocturnal sleep in normal young adults, whereas REM sleep takes place predominantly during the last third of the night's sleep.

The percentage of delta sleep is affected by age, amount of prior sleep, and various diseases. Delta sleep decreases with age and may be absent in healthy, elderly males. Sleep deprivation increases the rapidity of the onset of delta sleep and its portion of total sleep time.

Young children have particularly large proportions of delta sleep, which increases if they are sleep-deprived. This explains why it is frequently difficult to awaken children. Elderly people have smaller proportions of delta sleep, which is why they are easily aroused by environmental noise. Medical problems, such as obstructive sleep apnea, periodic leg movements during sleep, and fibromyalgia may affect quantity and quality of delta sleep. This in turn probably accounts in some measure for the feeling of fatigue experienced by people suffering from these maladies.

Fibromyalgia and Sleep

About twenty years ago, researchers in Toronto discovered that patients with fibromyalgia had NREM stages of sleep "contaminated" by an intercurrent alpha rhythm (like that of wakefulness). But whether the sleep disturbance caused the fibromyalgia symptoms or was secondary to the disease itself could not be determined.

This group of investigators went on to show that healthy subjects selectively deprived of delta sleep by being exposed to noise developed periods of delta sleep mixed with alpha waves. Interestingly, when deprived of delta sleep these people experienced some musculoskeletal discomfort and mood symptoms similar to those of the patients with fibromyalgia. These data suggested that the stage 4 sleep disturbance caused the appearance of the achiness or pain and mood symptoms.

However, it was felt that the effect of delta sleep disturbance on symptoms might be determined by examining the physical and psychological characteristics of the healthy subjects. Their subjects were younger than the patient population with fibromyalgia and free from illnesses and psychological problems, but they were not particularly physically fit. Yet they had the symptoms of fibromyalgia when put through the sleep-deprivation process. Their relatively sedentary lifestyle may have been significant, because most reports have pointed to the positive influence of exercise on delta sleep.

Sleep disturbances can be triggered in patients by physical or emotional trauma or by a metabolic or other medical problem. Poor sleep can lead to fatigue with resultant diminished exercise causing worsened physical fitness and the establishment of a vicious cycle of inactivity and sleep disturbance with physical and mood-related symptoms (see the Cycle of Inactivity on page 102). These problems could help lead to the development of fibromyalgia.

Hormones and Sleep

An interesting study published in the *Journal of Clinical Endocrinology and Metabolism* (April 2001) revealed that men seem to become more sensitive to the stimulating effects of *corticotropin-releasing hormone* (CRH) as they get older. This hormone plays a key role in how your body responds to stress. If you are aroused, you will have higher levels of CRH.

In the study, researchers evaluated the sleep habits of twelve middle-aged men and twelve young men over four nights. On one night, the men all received CRH ten minutes after they were asleep. Both groups of men produced higher levels of stress hormones in response to the CRH. While younger men produced higher levels of cortisol (the main stress hormone involved in the "fight or flight" response), middle-aged men stayed awake longer. They also had less slow-wave or deep sleep than did the younger men, showing that middle-aged men may have an increased vulnerability to stress hormones. This, in part, may explain why insomnia increases in middle age as a result of these dysfunctional sleep mechanisms caused by arousal-producing stress hormones. There are also studies showing that people who spend less time in slow-wave sleep are more prone to depression.

Because of the effects of estrogen on a woman's sleep pattern, it's more difficult to study women and sleep. Still, for those women who find it difficult to sleep during the premenstrual time, you have great company. Studies show that women have more awakenings, sleep disturbances, and vivid dreams during the premenstrual time than the rest of the month. Some women report having fatigue, no matter how long they stay in bed. Menstrual symptoms such as bloating, headache, abdominal cramps, food cravings, irritability, and emotional changes all appear to contribute to the inability to get sound sleep. These problems generally disappear a few days after menstruation begins.

For women in perimenopause or just prior to menopause, the declining levels of the hormone estradiol may increase your chance of poor sleep. In an intriguing study at the University of Pennsylvania Medical Center in Philadelphia published in *Obstetrics and Gynecology* (September 2001), researchers followed 436 women age thirty-five to forty-nine over a two-year period. About 17 percent of the women reported suffering from poor sleep throughout the entire study period. While researchers blamed anxiety, depression, and caffeine consumption as factors that disturbed the women's sleep, they also identified low estradiol levels and hot flashes in older women aged forty-five to forty-nine as responsible for the sleepless nights, even though all women were experiencing regular menstrual cycles and had not yet entered menopause. The study concluded that the decline in estradiol that occurs with ovarian aging might be associated with poor sleep in women. This sleep deprivation results in daytime fatigue and irritability and can even lead to feelings of depression—all symptoms of fibromyalgia syndrome, too.

These studies can help you to see the unique link between hormones, age, poor sleep, and the varied symptoms that can result. Use the information to assess your own bedtime habits and then use the suggestions on pages 201 to 203 to resolve your sleep problems associated with fibromyalgia.

ACCURATE DIAGNOSIS IS ESSENTIAL FOR PROPER THERAPY

Many of the symptoms that fibromyalgia patients experience are shared by those with other sleep disorders. For example, some patients with obstructive sleep apnea, intermittent blockages of the upper airway at the back of the tongue, which occurs in 2 percent of women and 4 percent of men who are thirty to sixty years old, also complain of unrefreshing sleep and "hurting all over" upon arising in the morning. They also have a history of snoring and other symptoms, including morning headaches, dry mouth, and an increased tendency to doze off during the day. Some patients with sleep apnea have high blood pressure.

If your doctor suspects that your sleep disorder may have a different cause, he or she may recommend that you have a sleep study. Sleep studies, called *polysomnography*, include an *electroencephalogram* (EEG), which measures the electrical activity of the brain, as well as the monitoring of oxygen levels, movements of chest wall and abdomen, and nasal and oral airflow. A sleep study may show apnea (periods without breathing), manifested by absent airflow at nose and mouth in conjunction with ongoing respiratory muscle efforts shown by movement of chest wall and abdomen. An apnea may cause decreases in blood oxygen levels. Sleep is often interrupted at the end of the apnea by awakening.

This breaking up of continuous sleep is a major cause of daytime fatigue and sleepiness. Periodic leg movements during sleep, also known as nocturnal myoclonus, may also be associated with alpha intrusions and are a common cause of sleep interruptions. These sleep disorders require specific therapy.

It should be noted that certain drug therapy for fibromyalgia may worsen obstructive sleep apnea and actually exacerbate the patient's symptoms of fatigue and restless sleep.

PSYCHOLOGICAL OUTCOME OF INSOMNIA AND SLEEP DEPRIVATION
Mood swings and irritability
Depression
Lack of patience
Intolerance
Forgetfulness
Difficulty learning
Decreased attention span
Negligence
Reduced performance

The Problem of Insomnia

Because patients with fibromyalgia have a specific type of insomnia, a disorder of initiating and/or maintaining sleep, it is important to apply certain treatment measures. Not only is attention to sleep hygiene important, but such stimulants as caffeine and nicotine must be avoided near bedtime. Regular daily exercise, including stretching and aerobic activity, is a form of treatment that can help to consolidate sleep and to alleviate other symptoms. Biofeedback and relaxation techniques, as discussed in chapter 7, are useful in overcoming problems of initiating sleep.

High levels of arousal associated with racing thoughts, worrying, or rumination may also delay sleep onset. Meditation or guided imagery (see chapter 7) can be used to help the patient relax while focusing thoughts on a neutral or enjoyable target.

Nutritional and Hormonal Therapy for Sleep Disorders

About forty years ago, pharmacological studies suggested that the hormone serotonin may have a role in sleep induction. Later on, experiments in animals showed that destruction of the parts of the brain that housed serotonin-containing nerve cells could produce total insomnia. Partial damage to these areas of the brain caused variable decreases in sleep. The percentage of destruction of these particular nerve cells was correlated with the amount of slow-wave sleep.

It turns out that a nutrient, an amino acid called *tryptophan,* is a precursor in the synthesis of serotonin in the brain. Since tryptophan is present in milk—and warm milk seems to help some individuals fall asleep—this amino acid became a popular item at health food stores as the home remedy for insomnia. However, some patients who ingested tryptophan as a dietary supplement developed a syndrome with features of a disease called *scleroderma,* which included skin tightening, pain in joints, muscle aches, and weakness. These patients also developed anxiety, depression, and difficulty learning. Some patients actually died. It was later thought that the deaths were due to a contaminant of tryptophan in the substance they took.

It needs to be pointed out that not everyone who took the drug experienced side effects. By the same token, not everyone experienced relief from insomnia. Tryptophan, needless to say, fell out of favor as a nutritional supplement and treatment for insomnia and was pulled off the shelves. As discussed in chapter 9, foods rich in carbohydrates can also boost serotonin levels in the brain, helping to induce feelings of sleepiness and relaxation.

Also, 5-HTP (see page 85), a derivative of the amino acid tryptophan, boosts serotonin in the body and has been shown in preliminary studies to relieve disordered sleep in some people.

Tips to Encourage Sleep

Establishing better sleep hygiene is vital in managing the symptoms of fibromyalgia. In our clinic, patients have experienced great success with the following suggestions:

Sleep only as much as needed to feel refreshed and healthy the following day, not more. Curtailing the time in bed seems to solidify sleep; excessively long times in bed seem related to fragmented and shallow sleep.

A regular arousal time in the morning strengthens circadian cycling and leads to regular times of sleep onset.

A steady daily amount of exercise probably deepens sleep; occasional exercise, however, does not necessarily improve sleep the following night.

Occasional loud noises (e.g., aircraft flyovers) disturb sleep even in people who are not awakened and cannot remember them in the morning. Sound-attenuated bedrooms may help those who must sleep close to noise.

Although excessively warm rooms disturb sleep, there is no evidence that an excessively cold room solidifies sleep.

Hunger may disturb sleep; a light carbohydrate snack before bedtime may help you avoid sleep disturbances.

Caffeine in the evening disturbs sleep, even in those who feel it does not.

Alcohol may help tense people fall asleep more easily, but ensuing sleep is then fragmented.

People who awake feeling angry and frustrated because they cannot sleep should not keep trying, but should turn on the light and do something different. You might have a light snack high in carbohydrates, read a book, or watch a television show in another room.

The chronic use of tobacco disturbs sleep.

Another procedure we use to help patients overcome conditioned insomnia is stimulus-control behavior therapy. The goal is to reassociate the bedroom stimuli with sleep rather than with frustration and arousal. To achieve this, patients are told that they are "misusing" their bed if they lie in it awake and frustrated. Richard Bootzin, the behavior therapist who initiated this approach, recommends the following rules:

Go to bed only when sleepy.

Use the bed only for sleeping; do not read, watch television, or eat in bed.

If unable to sleep, get up and move to another room. Stay up until you are really sleepy, then return to bed.

If sleep still does not come easily, get out of bed again. The goal is to associate bed with falling asleep quickly.

Set the alarm and get up at the same time each morning, regardless of how much you slept during the night. This helps the body acquire a constant sleep-wake rhythm.

Do not nap during the day.

If the above rules are followed, patients will usually sleep little during the first night. By the second or third night, patients are so tired that they fall asleep on the first or second attempt. Sleep patterns then fluctuate for a few weeks, but gradually the bedroom surroundings again become associated with sleep. However, most patients need a lot of encouragement during this difficult reconditioning period.

Precise diagnosis is essential to establish the existence of fibromyalgia and to distinguish this disease from other sleep disorders. Once the diagnosis is made, a multifaceted approach is then required to ensure restful and healing sleep and may require some combination of supportive psychotherapy, biofeedback-relaxation techniques, physical fitness training, antidepressants, or some other medicine as discussed in chapter 4, along with careful medical supervision by a physician.

9

STEP 6: FOLLOW THE NUTRITIONAL PLAN FOR HEALING

Although there are no specific "magic" foods that are proven to cure fibromyalgia, research has shown that there are some positive nutritional measures you can take to heal your body. Being at the proper weight and eating healthful foods, including those that are low in fat and high in immunity-boosting antioxidants and phytochemicals, work together to help maximize energy and alertness, while possibly minimizing the constant fatigue and lethargy that accompany this syndrome.

Maintaining health and feeling good becomes increasingly more complicated with chronic diseases like fibromyalgia. Good health is more about the precise balance of a sound body, mind, and spirit than just the absence of disease. There are unique links among the brain, the hormone system, and the immune system. Within this balance, these links make feeling our best a total experience—physical, mental, and emotional. Taking charge of the areas of your health that you *can* control helps to optimize how you feel even in the midst of the aches and fatigue of fibromyalgia.

Taking Control of Your Disease

Eating for wellness is one of the treatment areas that you do have control over. Knowing that you are doing all you can to eat healthily can give you a sense of power to sustain your physical needs and help you cope with the stresses of everyday life and fibromyalgia.

The food choices you make can affect your weight; obesity is a significant public health problem in the United States, as well as in other developed nations. Studies are now being conducted to see if obesity contributes to an impaired immune system. If this is the case, then it is even more necessary that everyone takes control of his or her weight and nutrition.

Nutrients Support Repair of the Body

Nutrients are special compounds found in foods that support the body's repair, growth, and wellness. They include vitamins, minerals, amino acids, essential fatty acids, and water, and the calorie sources of carbohydrate, protein, and fat. Some nutrients can be made by the body (nonessential nutrients) and others must come from the diet (essential nutrients). A deficiency of either type of nutrient may lead to illness if left untreated.

Antioxidants Give Cell Protection

Antioxidants are essential nutrients that help protect your body against life's stressors. Antioxidant food sources are rich in beta-carotene and vitamins C and E. Antioxidants are thought to play a role in the body's cell-protection system and to interfere with aging and the disease process by neutralizing highly reactive and unstable molecules, called free radicals, produced by the body. In research, free radicals have been shown to disrupt and tear apart vital cell structures like cell membranes. Antioxidants have been shown to tie up these free radicals and take away their destructive power, perhaps reducing the risk of a number of chronic diseases and even slowing the aging process. Eating for wellness requires a diet rich in antioxidants.

Some researchers think that antioxidants might help prevent damage in some types of arthritis and boost immune function when a system is under stress. Both are important benefits for patients.

UNDERSTANDING ANTIOXIDANT FOOD SOURCES

BETA-CAROTENE. Beta-carotene, found in apricots, carrots, cantaloupe, pumpkin, and spinach, is converted to vitamin A in the body. Because of a great deal of media attention, most people think of only beta-carotene as having antioxidant properties, but there are many other carotenoid compounds that do also, including:

alpha-carotene (found in carrots, cantaloupe, and pumpkin)
gamma-carotene (found in apricots and tomatoes)
beta-cryptoxanthin (found in mangoes, nectarines, peaches, and tangerines)
lycopene (found in guava, pink grapefruit, tomatoes, and watermelon)
lutein and zeaxanthin (found in beets, corn, and collard and mustard greens)

SOURCES OF BETA-CAROTENE

apricots	pumpkins
broccoli	red peppers
cantaloupes	spinach
carrots	sweet potatoes
collard greens	tomatoes
kale	turnip greens
papayas	winter squash
peaches	

VITAMIN C. Vitamin C (ascorbic acid) protects us against infection and aids in wound healing. When the body is under great stress, the blood levels of ascorbic acid have been found to decline. This decline also occurs with age in both men and women.

Vitamin C plays a vital role in boosting levels of the energizing brain chemical *norepinephrine*. Norepinephrine produces a feeling of alertness and increases concentration. A deficiency of vitamin C can therefore influence your mood as well, leaving you less attentive. It is essential to include plenty of vitamin C sources in your diet.

SOURCES OF VITAMIN C

broccoli	oranges
cantaloupes	peppers
grapefruit and	potatoes
grapefruit juice	strawberries
kiwi	tomatoes

VITAMIN E. Vitamin E is important to the body for the maintenance of cell membranes, and this vitamin's antioxidant effect may slow age-related changes in the body. There is now evidence that vitamin E plays a role in lowering the risk of coronary heart disease and heart attack. Adults with intestinal disorders of malabsorption may be deficient in vitamin E.

Because this vitamin is taken in through vegetables and seed oils, it is difficult to ingest large amounts, especially if you are following a low-fat diet.

If your diet is low in vitamin E food sources, check with your doctor and see if you should add 200 to 400 IU daily. Supplements can be found at grocery or health food stores and pharmacies.

SOURCES OF VITAMIN E

margarine	vegetable oils
nuts and seeds	wheat germ

Zinc to Resist Infection

Zinc also has antioxidant effects and is vital to the body's resistance to infection and for tissue repair. Many illnesses, such as some cancers, kidney disease, long-term infection, trauma, and cirrhosis of the liver, are associated with zinc deficiency.

Medications may also interfere with absorption in the intestines and cause a zinc deficiency.

More research infers that zinc can help to improve the immune system in elderly people. However, cautions must be raised as high doses of zinc are toxic and may, in fact, suppress the immune function. Again, check with your physician for what is safe in your situation.

Foods high in zinc include seafood, eggs, meats, whole grains, wheat germ, nuts, and seeds; tea and coffee may hinder absorption.

Magnesium to Reduce Pain

Magnesium is vital for healthy muscle metabolism and function. Yet, when you have a magnesium deficiency, you may experience excessive muscle tension, muscle spasms, restlessness, tics, and twitches. Studies now indicate that magnesium is particularly important for those with fibromyalgia as it inhibits nerve receptors linked to the trigger point pain and regulates the release of neurohormones.

In a comprehensive study published in the journal *Alternative Medicine Alert* (March 2002), researchers found that just 500 milligrams of oral magnesium taken daily can significantly increase muscle magnesium level and influence fibromyalgia symptoms. In another study published in the *Cochrane Database of Systematic Reviews* (2001), researchers found that magnesium supplementation can help to alleviate painful menstrual cramps, although they are unsure of the exact amount needed. Because magnesium supplementation can cause gastrointestinal symptoms, including watery diarrhea, talk to your doctor first before trying this therapy.

Foods high in magnesium include cereals, nuts, sunflower seeds, barley, quinoa, tofu, dairy products, bananas, pineapples, artichokes, avocados, lima beans, spinach, okra, hummus, oysters, mackerel, grouper, cod, and sole.

B Vitamins May Ease Your FMS Symptoms

There is strong indication that some foods high in the B vitamins help to alleviate some fibromyalgia symptoms. For instance, folic acid, a B vitamin, seems to be a leader in mood management. In research performed at Massachusetts General Hospital in Boston and the Baylor Research Institute in Dallas, studies conclude that people with low folic acid levels are more likely to have *melancholia*, a type of depression characterized by sadness and declines in mental and physical activity. The eight-week study of 213 patients also found that those with low levels of folic acid were significantly less likely to respond to treatment for depression with fluoxetine (Prozac), a common antidepressant medication used for fibromyalagia patients. Vitamin B_{12} works closely with folic acid to make red blood cells and prevent anemia, memory loss, nerve damage, muscle weakness, and fatigue. (If you are a vegetarian, getting ample vitamin B_{12} is difficult, so talk to your doctor to see if supplementation is necessary.)

Check out the following chart of the most healing B vitamins for fibromyalgia, and try to include some of these foods in your daily diet to help ease painful symptoms.

Food Sources of Therapeutic B Vitamins

Vitamin	Food Sources
B_1 (Thiamine)	Wheat germ, peanuts, peas
B_2 (Riboflavin)	Dairy products, broccoli, tuna, salmon
B_3 (Niacin)	Brewer's yeast, poultry, eggs, peanuts
B_6 (Pyridoxine)	Soybeans, liver, fish, bananas, oatmeal
B_{12} (Colabamine)	Oysters, eggs, dairy products
Folic acid	Green leafy vegetables, asparagus, cantaloupe, spinach, lima beans, kidney beans, pinto beans, navy beans, tofu, sweet potatoes, citrus fruits, peanuts
Biotin	Liver, nuts, legumes, egg yolks
Pantothenic acid	Cheese, cauliflower, beans, sweet potatoes

Choose Plant-Based Phytochemicals

Nutrition research is now revealing that a variety of food choices can do more than provide optimal nutrient intake. A varied diet can also provide hundreds of nutrient and nonnutrient compounds that may be vital to protection from disease. These compounds found in plant-based foods as a group are referred to as *phytochemicals*.

Phytochemicals appear in all plants. A diet that includes a variety of grains, fruits, and vegetables should provide these substances if you vary your choices and methods of food preparation. Although there are phytochemical supplements and pills, it is better to get your phytochemicals from a varied diet.

Tips to Boost Your Immune Power

- Use a tomato sauce over pasta
- Add tomato sauce to soups and stews
- Add sliced tomatoes to sandwiches and salads
- Add extra vegetables with antioxidants to your dishes
- Throw some greens and carrots in your vegetable soup
- Try a veggie pizza with broccoli and pepper
- Toss some grated zucchini into your next batch of muffins or load of bread
- Snack on dried fruits and nuts like apricots and cashews
- Use chopped nuts or wheat germ to top off your yogurt

Because of the wide array of nutrients in foods essential for wellness, including those not yet identified, relying on supplements for good nutrition may limit your intake to just known compounds.

A diet for wellness should contain foods loaded with phytochemicals.

PHYTOCHEMICAL FOOD SOURCES

PHYTOCHEMICAL	FOOD SOURCES	WELLNESS FACTOR
Carotenoids	Carrots, apricots, sweet potatoes	Prevent cancer and and heart disease
Indoles	Cruciferous vegetables like cabbage, broccoli, and cauliflower	Prevent breast and uterine cancer
Isoflavones	Legumes, soybeans	Prevent breast and uterine cancer
Lycopene	Tomatoes, red peppers, carrots	Prevent cancer
Sulfides (allyls)	Cabbage, onions broccoli, garlic, brussels sprouts	Prevent cancer

Other Immune Boosters

A great concern to anyone with a chronic illness is avoiding other illnesses. For example, fibromyalgia can make you feel flulike with the muscle aches and fatigue. So getting the flu on top of having fibromyalgia is like a double whammy. What about those who have fibromyalgia and also develop osteoporosis or heart disease? It doesn't have to happen to you, and one way to protect yourself from viruses, infections, and other chronic illnesses is to keep your immune system boosted so it can adequately fight to keep you well.

FLAVONOIDS

Flavonoids (or bioflavonoids) include about four thousand compounds that are responsible for the colors of fruits and flowers. Hosts of experiments on bioflavonoids found in the soft white skin of citrus fruits have suggested that these key nutrients increase immune system activation. These biochemically active substances accompany vitamin C in plants and act as an antioxidant. You can find bioflavonoids in grapefruit, oranges, lemons, and limes. Rose hips, apricots, cherries, grapes, black currants, plums, blackberries, and papayas are other fruit sources of bioflavonoids. Green peppers, broccoli, eggplant, squash, and tomatoes are some good vegetable sources of bioflavonoids. Tea, red wine, and parsley are also good sources.

QUERCETIN

This is a very highly concentrated form of bioflavonoids that is found in citrus fruits, red and yellow onions, and broccoli. Quercetin reduces inflammation associated with allergies and can inhibit the growth of head and neck cancers. Other citrus flavonoids include *hesperidin,* which is said to raise blood levels of the "good" high-density lipoprotein (HDL fats) and lower the "bad" low-density lipoprotein (LDL fats) and triglycerides, and *tangeritin,* which induces apoptosis, or programmed cell death, in leukemia cells, but does not harm normal cells.

GLUTATHIONE

Another nutrient that has been found to strengthen the immune system so it can fight other infections is glutathione. This powerful antioxidant is most plentiful in the red, pulpy area of the watermelon near the rind. It can also be found in cruciferous vegetables.

Five a Day

As you learn to eat for wellness, it is important to follow the nutritional recommendations from the USDA (United States Department of Agriculture), which advises eating five servings of fruits and vegetables a day. Through groundbreaking research, this organization has concluded that we are what we eat, and the nutritional components of fruits and vegetables can prevent or even reverse some diseases and conditions. The National Cancer Institute goes one step beyond the USDA's recommendation by encouraging us to eat nine servings of fruits and vegetables (or more) a day for better health.

Adding Phytochemicals to Your Diet

- Use spinach, shredded cabbage, sliced carrots, and broccoli in your salads
- Add chopped fruits to cereal, yogurt, ice cream, and muffins
- Snack on cut-up carrots, pepper, broccoli, and cauliflower
- Make a quick dip by adding tomato salsa to nonfat yogurt
- Fill your pantry with plenty of herbs and spices like ginger, garlic, chives, and parsley
- Frequently include steamed cabbage, broccoli, or brussels sprouts with meals

---

Whether you opt for five a day or can reach the ultimate goal of nine servings a day, it is important to know why this recommendation is important to maintaining good health. The answer lies in the ability of these food sources to prevent a wide range of chronic diseases and bolster the body's immune power. They provide the basic elements for a healthful diet as high-fiber, low-fat powerhouses of antioxidants and phytochemicals, among many other essential and nonessential nutrients.

EASY WAYS TO ADD FRUITS AND VEGETABLES TO YOUR DAILY DIET

Breakfast:	4 oz. of grapefruit juice (1)
	1 bagel with jelly
	½ cup skim milk
Snack:	1 cup low-fat yogurt
	½ cup raspberries (1)
Lunch:	½ cup spinach salad (1)
	tuna sandwich with a sliced tomato (1)
	1 cup skim milk

Dinner: ½ cup broccoli (1)
                           4 oz. baked chicken breast
                           ½ cup wild rice
                           rolls
                           ½ cup sherbet

TOTAL FOR DAY: Five servings of fruits and vegetables

To meet the goal for nine fruits and vegetables a day, increase the amount of salad, vegetables, fruits, and juice to reach the total.

Eat Frequently to Boost Energy

Many FMS patients have found that eating frequent mini-meals helps in keeping energy levels higher and also helps to maintain a normal weight. Studies show that eating *more frequently* throughout the day, as opposed to three heavy meals, will boost your metabolism and productivity. Research has found that people who eat two meals or less during the day have a slower metabolic rate (the speed at which your body burns calories, and the rate that we all want to go faster) versus those who eat three or more times a day.

Eating frequent meals that are high in complex carbohydrates (fruits, vegetables, and whole grains) and protein will also keep your blood glucose constant so you do not feel irritable or overly hungry. When you eat refined carbohydrates that have been processed, they can raise your blood sugar quickly and can leave you feeling fatigued. A diet that is low in protein may cause you to feel drowsy. Eating complex carbs and proteins together at each mini-meal helps to slow absorption, giving you more staying power and keeping blood sugar levels more even.

An easy way to adjust to mini-meals is to break your daily food intake into five or six small meals, spaced every three to four hours throughout the day. Each mini-meal will have about three hundred to four hundred calories. You can adjust these, depending on your total caloric goal.

Your daily menu may look like this:

Mini-meal 1: 1 cup yogurt, 6 oz. juice, 1 slice toast, hot tea

Mini-meal 2: 2 wheat crackers with 1 Tbsp. peanut butter, ½ cup strawberries

Mini-meal 3: 3 oz. water-packed tuna, low-fat mayo, lettuce, tomato, 2 slices bread, 1 apple, tea

Mini-meal 4: ½ banana spread with 1 Tbsp. peanut butter, ½ cup skim milk

Mini-meal 5: 3 oz. baked skinless chicken breast, 1 baked potato with low-fat sour cream, 1 cup steamed broccoli, mineral water

Mini-meal 6: 3 cups air-popped popcorn, ½ cup red grapes

Select Foods Low on the Glycemic Index

If you have a problem with feelings of fatigue and irritability between meals, it could be related to blood glucose fluctuations. I recommend that some patients try to follow the glycemic index (GI), if blood glucose fluctuations keeps them from feeling their best. The glycemic index represents a numerical system of measuring how fast a carbohydrate food triggers a rise in circulating blood sugar two to three hours after eating. Fats and protein foods do not cause a dramatic rise or fall in blood glucose levels. Yet carbohydrates do, and the higher the number, the greater the blood sugar response. For instance, if a carbohydrate food is low on the glycemic index, there might be a small rise in blood sugar; a food high on the index may trigger a more dramatic rise.

I find this index beneficial as it helps patients to monitor what they eat each day and gives them some control in diminishing fatigue, particularly the feelings of weakness and inability to concentrate you might experience when your blood sugar levels drop between meals.

GO!

SELECT FOODS LOW ON THE GLYCEMIC INDEX
Fruits
Vegetables (low starch)

Low-fat dairy, including yogurt
Low-fat protein and legumes
Nuts and seeds
Soy products
Unrefined grains (whole grain)

CAUTION!
CHOOSE FEWER FOODS HIGH ON THE GLYCEMIC INDEX
Cookies, candy, pastries
Pasta
Potatoes
Refined grains
Rice
Vegetables (high starch)

Add Dietary Fiber to Daily Meal Plan

Dietary fiber is one more valuable bonus we get from eating five to nine (or more) servings of fruits and vegetables per day. It is the part of the plant that we can eat but our bodies cannot digest or break down. Fiber moves foods and the toxins they contain quickly through the digestive tract, allowing less time for any possible cancer-causing agents to come in contact with the intestines, colon, or rectum. According to the National Cancer Institute, a diet high in fiber cuts the risk of colon cancer by up to 70 percent and may also lower the risk of kidney stones and gallstones, as well as ease constipation. Fiber ferments in the colon, increasing the amount of oxygen, which in turn diminishes the action of the harmful bacteria. Fresh, whole fruits and vegetables, including the skins, provide the most benefit from fiber. Figs, prunes, and dried beans and peas are also very high in fiber, so include them in the diet on a regular basis.

The National Cancer Institute recommends 25 to 35 grams of fiber per day, yet most Americans eat considerably less than that. About one-fourth of your daily fiber intake should consist of the soluble type fiber found in oats, beans, fruits, and vegetables.

The rest of your fiber intake should come from the insoluble type, found in wheat bran and whole grains.

FOODS HIGH IN SOLUBLE FIBER

acorn squash	dates
apples	dried beans
baked potatoes	lentils
blueberries	peas
broccoli	prunes
cabbage	pumpkins
carrots	raspberries
cauliflower	strawberries
citrus fruits	sweet potatoes

You can increase your dietary fiber by adding at least six servings of whole grain breads and cereals, pasta, rice, and dried peas and beans, along with the five to nine servings of fruits and vegetables, to your diet. As you begin to include low-fat, high–complex carbohydrate foods in your diet, you will notice a gradual reduction in your weight. For most patients, this is an appreciated added benefit.

GUIDELINES TO INCREASE FIBER

Eat more legumes that are very high in fiber. Red beans, black beans, great northern beans, and other legumes are high in fiber and have no fat. Don't cook legumes with animal fat.

Eat raw vegetables for snacks. Two carrots will give you a day's supply of vitamin A and provide more than 7 grams of fiber.

Read your cereal box at the grocery store. If the cereal has less than 3 grams of fiber, it probably has little nutrient value.

The Fiber Content of Selected Foods (Grams)

1 medium bran muffin	3
1 slice of whole wheat toast	2
1 ounce of raisin bran	4
⅔ cup of oatmeal	4.5
1 medium apple with skin	3
1 medium orange	3
1 medium raw carrot	4
½ cup of cooked kidney beans	7

Add dried fruits to your cereal. Three prunes can give you 4 grams of fiber.

Keep your vegetables crisp when you cook them. Eat them with skins on to add to the fiber content.

Eat fruits with the skin on for an extra fiber boost.

Top Ten Power Healers

It's important that each food choice be high in healing nutrients to feel your best with fibromyalgia. I recommend that patients try to include the following healing foods in their daily diet, as these are known to be super-healers. I've given you a sample recipe for each food to show you how a bit of creativity goes a long way in optimizing taste and nutrition. You can also use the following ideas:

Sauté broccoli sprouts with fresh garlic in olive oil.
Add tomato slices to a lunchtime tuna sandwich.
Drink low-fat milk with your meals.
Have a quick snack of soy nuts and hot green tea.
Freeze grapes and enjoy as a snack on a warm summer day.

BROCCOLI

This green, treelike vegetable is full of indoles, isothiocyanates, and sulforaphane—phytochemicals that pack a power punch of healing nutrition! If you really want the highest concentration of these cancer-fighting compounds, get broccoli sprouts at your local health food store. The sprouts have ten to a hundred times more sulforaphane than mature broccoli.

Lemon Almond Broccoli

1 16-ounce package of frozen broccoli (or use 1 bunch fresh)
2 tablespoons butter
1 tablespoon lemon juice
½ cup slivered almonds
salt and pepper to taste

To make:
Preheat oven to 325 degrees; lightly grease a 1½-quart baking dish. Cook broccoli according to directions, drain, and spoon into the baking dish. Squeeze lemon over the broccoli. Melt butter, and pour over the dish. Top with almonds and a dash of salt and pepper. Bake at 325 degrees for 15 minutes.

Makes 4 servings.

DAIRY PRODUCTS

Low-fat dairy products such as low-fat milk, buttermilk, cheese and cheese products, cottage cheese, ice milk, and yogurt are all important in keeping your body functioning at its peak. The calcium and vitamin D in dairy products help to keep bones strong and prevent osteoporosis and fractures. Studies show that a diet high in low-fat dairy products and fruits and vegetables significantly lowers blood pressure.

Orange Yogurt Dip

   4 ounces light cream cheese, softened
   2 tablespoons confectioners sugar
   1 8-ounce container low-fat vanilla yogurt
   1 teaspoon orange zest
   ¼ teaspoon grated ginger (or ginger powder)
   ½ teaspoon vanilla flavoring
   Assorted seasonal fruit to dip: strawberries, apples, or
      melons

To make:
In medium bowl, combine cream cheese and powdered sugar.
Mix until creamy, slowly adding yogurt, orange zest, and ginger.
Beat until fluffy and chill in refrigerator for 1 hour. Serve with
assorted seasonal fruit. Cut slivers of orange peel for decora-
tion, and place along the edge of the tray.

Makes 6 to 8 servings.

FISH

New studies show that eating fish at least once a week can cut
the risk of sudden cardiac death. One eleven-year study of
20,551 male physicians found that men who ate fish once a week
had half the risk of sudden cardiac death as those who ate fish
less than once a month. Although this study focused on men, it
wouldn't hurt women to get on the bandwagon! Substances in
fish called omega-3 fatty acids may have a protective effect
against sudden cardiac death, possibly by preventing potentially
dangerous arrhythmias or irregular heartbeats. Some heart-
healthy fish include anchovies, bluefish, lobster, mackerel, salmon,
sardines, scallops, tuna, and whitefish.

Tuna Salad Pitas

9 ounces white chunk tuna packed in distilled or spring
    water, drained, and flaked
¼ cup thin sliced onion
½ cup diced seeded cucumber, unpeeled
¼ cup plus 2 tablespoons fat-free, cholesterol-free or light,
    reduced-calorie mayonnaise dressing
¼ cup sliced green onions
2 teaspoons grated ginger root
½ apple, thinly sliced
1 tablespoon finely snipped fresh cilantro
½ teaspoon grated lemon zest
dash of red hot-pepper sauce
5 six-inch whole wheat pita breads
5 small pieces of leaf lettuce

To make:
In a medium bowl, combine tuna salad ingredients. Cover and
refrigerate until thoroughly chilled, at least 30 minutes. Split
each pita carefully around the top edge, about one third of the
circumference of the bread. Put lettuce leaf and about ½ cup
tuna mixture in each pita.

Makes 5 servings.

GARLIC

Scientific research claims that garlic contains chemicals that act
like ACE (angiotensin-converting enzyme) inhibitors, those
prescription drugs commonly given to lower blood pressure and
protect the heart. Supplements of garlic reduce blood pressure
by dilating blood vessels. In fact, some studies have revealed
that ingesting as much as one or two cloves of fresh garlic per
day can lower mild blood pressure an average of 8 percent in
one to three months. Researchers have found that garlic and
onions can block formation of nitrosamines. These are powerful

carcinogens that target several sites in the body, usually the liver, colon, and breasts.

Roasted Garlic Humus

1 whole head garlic
1 15-ounce can garbanzo (chickpeas) beans, drained
¼ pound firm tofu, drained
2 tablespoons fresh lemon juice
1 tablespoon olive oil
½ teaspoon ground cumin
¼ teaspoon salt
1 tablespoon fresh cilantro, minced

To make:
Preheat oven to 350 degrees. Remove white skin from garlic head. Do not peel or separate the cloves. Wrap garlic in foil, and bake at 350 degrees for one hour. Remove from oven and cool. Separate cloves, and squeeze garlic pulp into food processor. Discard skins.

Add drained garbanzos, tofu, lemon juice, olive oil, cumin, and salt to the garlic pulp. Process until smooth. Transfer the mixture to a bowl, and sprinkle cilantro on top. Serve with tortilla chips or pita wedges.

GREEN TEA

Green tea is a powerful antioxidant and may help in reducing the risk of cardiovascular disease and stroke. Some new studies indicate that it may help in preventing osteoporosis, and other findings reveal that it may help to prevent pancreatic, breast, lung, esophageal, and skin cancers. Researchers report that a nontoxic chemical found in green tea, *epigallocatechin-3 gallate,* acts against *urokinase* (an enzyme crucial for cancer growth). One cup of green tea contains between 100 and 200 milligrams of the antitumor ingredient.

Green Tea Refresher

3 cups freshly brewed green tea (follow package directions)
1 cup fresh blueberries
1 cup fresh orange and apple slices
1 cup cranberry juice
1 cup pineapple juice
1 cup ginger ale

To make:
Combine cranberry juice, pineapple juice, and fruit in a saucepan. Bring these ingredients to a boil, and then turn off the unit. When cool, pour this combination into a large pitcher. Add the green tea, ginger ale, and 2 cups crushed ice. Sweeten with sugar or honey, if preferred.

Makes around 2 quarts.

OLIVE OIL

Olive oil is a mono-unsaturated fat that has also been promoted recently as a heart-healthy oil that is preferable to other vegetable oils and margarine. In Mediterranean countries, olive oil is widely used both for cooking and as a salad oil. Breast cancer rates are also 50 percent lower in those countries than in the United States.

Jalapeño Basil Slaw with Olive Oil Dressing

2 cups shaved green cabbage
2 cups shaved red cabbage
1 red onion, sliced thin
1 julienne carrot
2 seeded and julienne jalapeños
½ cup coarsely chopped cilantro leaves

For the vinaigrette dressing:
1 cup loosely packed basil leaves (fresh)
1 shallot, chopped
2 cloves garlic
½ cup light olive oil
2 teaspoons honey
¼ cup rice vinegar
1 teaspoon salt
¼ teaspoon black pepper

To make:
Mix together cabbages, onion, carrot, jalapeños, and cilantro. Chill until ready to serve. In a blender, place basil, shallot, garlic, and olive oil. Blend until smooth. Transfer to bowl and add honey, vinegar, and salt and pepper. Pour over slaw just before serving, and toss.

Serves 6 to 8.

RED GRAPES
A new super antioxidant, called activin, has been discovered inside the seeds of red grapes. By-products of the red grape, such as wine, juice, or seeds, may offer significant protection against certain types of cancer, heart disease, rheumatoid arthritis, cataracts, and many other chronic and degenerative diseases. Some studies show that activin is up to seven times more powerful as an antioxidant than vitamins C, E, and beta-carotene. This may explain why red wine is more healthful than white wine in protecting you from heart disease. Recent studies conclude that a glass of wine a day may also reduce the risk of age-associated vision loss.

Mandarin Orange-Grape Spinach Salad

4 cups fresh spinach, cleaned and dried
1 small can mandarin oranges, drained
½ cup red grapes, sliced in half
2 tablespoons red onion, chopped
¼ cup sunflower seeds

Dressing

You need:
½ cup orange juice
1 tablespoon extra light olive oil

To make:
Arrange spinach leaves on four individual plates. Spoon the mandarin oranges, grapes, red onions, and sunflower seeds on top of each salad, dividing equally. To make vinaigrette: In a small bowl combine orange juice and olive oil and whisk, pouring over each salad.

Makes 4 servings.

SOY
There is some new evidence that a soy-based diet may reduce pain and inflammation, which is potentially good news for those who suffer with fibromyalgia and other arthritis-related diseases. The research, presented in March 2001 at the American Pain Society meeting in Baltimore, Maryland, concluded that rats who were fed a soy protein diet experienced significantly less pain and swelling than rats who received a milk-protein diet. In the study, investigators at Johns Hopkins gave the rats either a placebo or a solution that caused inflammation to build up in the rat's hind paw. After a period of time, rats on the soy-protein diet were able to tolerate more pain than the milk-protein group. Of course, this study was done on animals and it

will be a while before we can conclude the same for human beings. Nonetheless, the future is bright for alternative therapies to treat pain and inflammation, and studies like this open the door to new treatments.

Vegetarians have known for years that soy protein is an easy, inexpensive, and healthful alternative to meat. Soy products are dairy-free and do not contain saturated fat. For years, soybeans have played an integral part in Asian culture. In fact, heart disease, breast cancer, prostate cancer, and osteoporosis rates for Asian men and women are much lower than for Americans. In a recent study of one thousand people reported in the *American Journal of Epidemiology* (December 1, 1996), those who ate soybeans in some form at least once a week had half the risk of developing the polyps that are precursors to colon cancer compared to those who did not eat soybeans.

Isoflavones are phytonutrients found in soy that are converted into phytoestrogens (plant estrogens that are close in structure to the body's form of estrogen) in the body. Although these plant ingredients mimic the hormone estrogen, they appear to have no harmful side effects and can relieve menopausal symptoms that frequently occur because of plummeting estrogen levels. Studies show that soy protein isolate can also effectively prevent the rise in serum cholesterol associated with ovarian hormone deficiency. If you want to increase soy in your diet yet aren't fond of tofu, try such soy-based products as meatless pepperoni, salami, hot dogs, bacon, puddings, and dairy alternatives. Some calcium-rich soy foods include tahini, calcium-set tofu, fortified soy milk, textured vegetable protein, and soy nuts.

Tofu Crumble Chili

1 large onion, chopped
1 large bell pepper, chopped
2 tablespoons olive oil
1 12-ounce package of prebrowned, all-vegetable-protein
   crumbles (tofu) (frozen)
2 cups water or low-sodium broth
4 16-ounce cans diced tomatoes with garlic and onions
   (or favorite)
2 15-ounce cans dark kidney beans (drained)
2 cups soybeans, cooked, drained (optional)
½ teaspoon Salt Free Garlic and Herb Seasoning
   (McCormick)
½ teaspoon onion powder
1 teaspoon chili powder
½ teaspoon red pepper
1 tablespoon Worcestershire sauce
salt and pepper, to taste
1 4-ounce can chilies (optional)
2 tablespoons fresh cilantro, chopped
½ cup fat-free or light sour cream (optional)

To make:
In a large soup pot, sauté chopped onion and pepper in olive oil
on medium high heat for 3 to 4 minutes. Add tofu crumbles,
and cook 4 minutes longer. Add water or broth, tomatoes,
drained kidney beans, soybeans, spices, Worcestershire sauce
and chilies. Adjust spices; add salt and pepper to taste. Cover
and cook on low for 2 hours to thicken sauce. Add cilantro just
before serving; serve over brown rice. Top each bowl of Tofu
Crumble Chili with a dollop of sour cream and a sprinkle of
cheese.

Makes 12 servings.

SPINACH

Homocysteine has been a big news maker. This naturally occurring blood protein promotes artery clogging and is a by-product of meals high in protein. How do you counteract homocysteine? Add more folic acid. Folic acid, which is found in spinach, dramatically lowers elevated levels of homocysteine in the blood. Age-related macular degeneration (AMD), the leading cause of blindness in older people, is also significantly decreased by eating this green vegetable. Spinach is high in folacin, a nutrient crucial during early pregnancy to prevent neural-tube defects in children, and this power vegetable is also rich in beta-carotene, vitamins A and C, and potassium. You can easily get the minimum daily intake of folate (400 mcg) by adding the following to your diet:

Dark green vegetables
Fruits, especially citrus fruits or juices
Whole grains
Enriched breakfast cereals

Fresh Spinach-Orzo Salad

4 cups fresh spinach, cleaned and dried
½ cup black olives, pitted and sliced
3 green onions, diced
¼ cup sun-dried tomatoes (in oil, drained)
½ cucumber, diced
1 cup cooked and drained orzo pasta
¼ cup toasted pine nuts or walnuts
¼ cup fresh grated Parmesan cheese

To make:
Put the spinach in a large bowl and, using kitchen scissors, cut it into very tiny pieces. Add the sliced olives, diced green onion, sun-dried tomatoes, and diced cucumber. Toss the vegetables with the cooked orzo, nuts, and Parmesan cheese. Add your favorite vinaigrette when ready to serve.

Makes 4 servings.

TOMATOES

Preliminary research confirms that the potent antioxidant lycopene, which is prominent in tomatoes, may be more powerful than beta-carotene, alpha-carotene, and vitamin E. This antioxidant is associated with protection against heart disease and certain cancers such as prostate and lung cancer. Cooking tomatoes releases the lycopene and makes it available for absorption in your body.

Mediterranean Garbanzos and Tomatoes

4 tablespoons extra virgin olive oil
1 medium red onion, chopped
4 cloves garlic, minced
2 cans garbanzo beans (chickpeas), rinsed and drained
2 ripe tomatoes, chopped
1 cucumber, thinly sliced
⅓ cup fresh basil, shredded
½ cup Parmesan cheese, shredded
¼ cup balsamic vinegar
1 teaspoon sugar
¼ teaspoon crushed red pepper flakes

To make:
Heat 2 tablespoons of the oil in large skillet. Add onion and garlic; cook 5 minutes while stirring. Add garbanzo beans to onion and garlic; cook and stir 5 minutes until heated. Spoon mixture onto a large serving platter. Top beans with tomatoes, cucumber slices, and basil. Drizzle with a dressing made from remaining 2 tablespoons olive oil, balsamic vinegar, sugar, and crushed red pepper flakes. Serve warm or at room temperature on a bed of romaine or favorite lettuce.

Serves 4 to 6.

Foods for a Calming Effect

As we have discussed above, good nutrition influences our ability to stay healthy and recent research has revealed that what we eat can affect our moods as well. In the past twenty years, hundreds of studies have confirmed a connection between certain foods and our ability to feel calm and alert. Dr. Judith Wurtman, a nutrition researcher at the Massachusetts Institute of Technology, has found that certain foods affect brain chemicals that influence our mood, mental energy, and performance.

These "persuasive" foods are high in carbohydrates, such as breads, cereal, pasta, or sherbet, and raise the level of serotonin in the brain. When serotonin levels rise, we feel calm and upbeat for a period of time. As discussed throughout the book, serotonin is the mood-elevating neurotransmitter; it plays an unknown role in fibromyalgia symptoms, especially with depression and sleep disorders. Studies have shown that by including plenty of foods high in complex carbohydrates in your diet, you can boost the level of serotonin and reap the benefits of feeling calm throughout the day and sleeping more soundly at night.

Even though we have a host of new information on the food-mood connection, finding foods that relieve depressed feelings relies on a personal trial-and-error approach. Using the list of the suggested serotonin-boosting foods below, see which ones make a difference in your symptoms and wellness, and then incorporate these in five to six mini-meals throughout the day to keep blood sugar and energy levels even.

HIGH-CARBOHYDRATE FOODS THAT BOOST SEROTONIN

bagels	pasta
bread	potatoes
cereal	rice
crackers	sherbet
muffins	

Foods to Boost Energy and Alertness

Just as some foods can be used to create a calm feeling during times when you experience great stress or anxiety, other foods can create the opposite effect, making you feel attentive and responsive. Foods rich in protein, like turkey, tuna, or chicken, are also rich in an amino acid called tyrosine. Tyrosine boosts levels of the neurotransmitters dopamine and norepinephrine. Neurotransmitters are the chemicals that send messages from cell to cell. Sophisticated research by Dr. Judith Wurtman at the Massachusetts Institute of Technology has revealed that people are more alert when the brain is producing the neurotransmitters dopamine and norepinephrine. The neurotransmitter serotonin is associated with less anxiety and increased drowsiness. Dopamine and norepinephrine may be produced through the dietary consumption of protein. When we eat protein food, this increases the amino acid tyrosine, which boosts the levels of dopamine and norepinephrine. This, in turn, creates a feeling of alertness and improves our concentration. A protein source should be included in your diet several times a day, especially during those times when you need to clear your mind and boost your energy.

Try the following to see which foods boost stamina and alertness.

HIGH-PROTEIN FOODS RICH IN TYROSINE

beef	soy products
cheese	(soybeans, soy
fish	granules, soy
legumes and peas	milk, etc.)
milk	yogurt
poultry	

Repairing the Damage of Fibromyalgia

Protein is also important in building and repairing body tissue and in fighting infection. Too little protein in the diet may lead to symptoms of fatigue, weakness, apathy, and poor immunity. The average-size adult needs 45 to 55 grams of protein a day. More protein is needed if there is fever or infection.

One ounce of meat, chicken, cheese, or fish provides 7 grams of protein; 1 cup of milk provides 8 grams of protein. Therefore 5 to 6 ounces of meat per day and 2 cups of milk provide adequate protein for most adults. Vegetable proteins can make a good substitute for animal protein, if eaten with a complementary starch at the same meal. An example of this would be to substitute 1½ cups of black beans and rice for a 2-ounce portion of meat.

COMPLEMENTARY VEGETABLE PROTEINS
beans and bread
beans and rice
corn tortillas and beans
legumes and grains
peanut butter and bread

Include Iron-Rich Foods

Some specific nutrient deficiencies can impact on how you feel. For example, if you are not including iron-rich foods in your diet (especially menstruating women), then iron-deficiency anemia can result. Symptoms of fatigue, weakness, shortness of breath, and pallor can compound symptoms of fibromyalgia. Make sure your diet includes plenty of iron-rich foods.

IRON-RICH FOODS
dried apricots
dried beans
enriched or fortified bread and cereals

lean, fat-trimmed cuts of red meat (beef, veal, or lamb)
lentils
prunes
raisins

When eating an iron-rich food from a plant source, include a vitamin C source, such as orange or grapefruit juice, along with it to enhance iron absorption. Vitamin C-fortified apple juice is also a good source.

Minimize PMS with Nutritional and Activity Changes

Because female patients with fibromyalgia tend to suffer with painful menstrual cramps, it is important to minimize premenstrual syndrome (PMS) symptoms through some dietary and activity changes. PMS symptoms may include mild breast tenderness, fluid retention, anxiety, dietary cravings, irritability, and an inability to concentrate. Unfortunately, neither the cause nor the cure for PMS is currently known. However, these measures may help alleviate some of the symptoms.

Eat a balanced diet that includes a variety of complex carbohydrate foods (grains, fruits, and vegetables) and a moderate amount of meat and milk products.

Exercise regularly to reduce stress and keep your body fit. A daily exercise program can decrease PMS symptoms. This lessening of symptoms may be connected with the rise in endorphins that occurs with an intense aerobic workout. Regular aerobic exercise increases one's sense of well-being and decreases fluid retention. It has also been shown to be effective in the treatment of depression.

Avoid alcohol before your menstrual period. Since alcohol is a mood-altering drug, it can compound feelings

of depression and hopelessness. Furthermore, many women have a decreased tolerance for alcohol prior to their period, and they may become intoxicated quickly.

Avoid caffeine before and during your menstrual period. Studies have shown that symptoms of PMS increase with the consumption of caffeine-containing beverages. In one study, women who totally abstained from caffeine had a complete resolution of symptoms from PMS.

Reduce excessive sodium and salt in the diet to reduce fluid retention. Excessive sodium can lead to bloating, edema, and fluid weight gain during premenstruation; reducing the sodium in the diet can relieve some of these symptoms. The best approach is to eat more foods naturally low in sodium. This includes fresh fruits and vegetables, cereals, and grains. Another way is to limit the consumption of high-sodium processed foods and the use of table salt. You can add a splash of lemon juice to a glass of water for a natural diuretic.

If you experienced premenstrual symptoms of *hypoglycemia* (low blood sugar), such as fatigue, dizziness, and the shakes, divide your meals into six small minimeals rich in complex carbohydrates and protein and low in simple sugars.

FOODS HIGH IN SIMPLE SUGARS
cakes
candy and gum
canned fruits in syrup
cookies
frozen yogurt and sherbet
fruit juice
pies
regular sodas and sweetened drinks

FOODS HIGH IN SODIUM

canned meats

canned soups

canned tomato products

canned vegetables

frozen prepared meals (vegetables with sauces, meats, casseroles)

processed meats

salted snacks, such as chips, peanuts, pretzels

Vitamin Supplements

Various vitamins and minerals have also been suggested as effective for treatment of chronic muscle pain. No specific evidence favors any single vitamin or mineral supplement, but if you are in doubt, talk with your physician or licensed nutritionist. Premenopausal women especially need to check for iron deficiency. Even a mild deficiency in iron can make it difficult to get through the day without overwhelming fatigue.

If you do take vitamins to boost your immune power, start with a multiple vitamin without minerals that has the Recommended Dietary Allowance (RDA) as suggested by the American Dietetics Association, and then talk with a nutritionist about your specific vitamin needs.

Omega-3

Some foods have been shown to decrease inflammation in the body, whereas others tend to increase the possibility of inflammation. For example, animal foods contain fats that have been found to increase an inflammatory response. But studies show that eating high-fat fish, such as mackerel, bluefish, or tuna, that contain omega-3 fatty acids enables the body to make products that tend to decrease the inflammation.

The most commonly available of these omega-3 fatty acids is found in some fish and fish oil. Although guidelines have not been established regarding supplements of fish oil, EPA (eicos-apentaenoic acid) is available in capsules without a prescription. You can ask for these capsules at your drugstore or health food store. Check the instructions on the label as to suggested dosage.

Some patients with arthritis have found improvement in pain and stiffness when they take these capsules for a few months. It is important to use EPA in addition to your basic treatment program, not in replacement of it. When used in the dosage prescribed on the label, no serious side effects are known.

Vegetarians who want to gain this anti-inflammatory benefit can substitute borage seed oil, flaxseed oil, black currant seed oil (BCSO), or evening primrose oil—all said to be helpful in offsetting the inflammation caused by arthritis. These oils all contain gammalinolenic acid (GLA), an omega-6 oil. One study of patients with active rheumatoid arthritis found that BCSO is a potentially effective treatment. Similar studies with fibromyalgia patients have not yet been conclusive.

FISH HIGH IN OMEGA-3

anchovies	salmon
bluefish	sardines
capeline	shad
dogfish	sturgeon
herring	tuna
mackerel	whitefish

The Fibromyalgia Food Elimination Diet

Over the years, I've found that food plays a key role in the symptoms some patients feel. When they eliminate one or more foods from their daily diet, the fibromyalgia symptoms subside. In an interesting study presented in October 2001 at the American College of Nutrition in Orlando, Florida, researchers reviewed the medical charts of seventeen fibromyalgia patients who eliminated foods such as corn, wheat, dairy, citrus, and soy from their diets. After two weeks, nearly half of the volunteers reported a significant reduction of pain and 76 percent also had a reduction in other FMS symptoms such as bloating, heartburn, breathing difficulties, and fatigue.

After the elimination phase of the study, participants then reintroduced specific foods every two to three days. They also monitored their reactions to the foods. The most common offenders were dairy, citrus, corn, wheat, and sugar, resulting in such symptoms as gastrointestinal distress, headache, or overall pain.

While this study is in its preliminary stages, it may benefit other FMS patients who are willing to try a restrictive diet to see if they can identify any food triggers.

Getting Started on the Elimination Diet

PHASE 1—ELIMINATION

Eliminate the following foods for two weeks. Be sure to read the labels of packaged foods to see if any of the following are listed in the ingredients:

milk (butter, ice cream, yogurt, cheese, and other by-products)

wheat (all breads, crackers, cookies, noodles, and other by-products)

corn (grits, popcorn, corn chips, corn syrups, corn starches, and by-products)

citrus (oranges, grapefruits, lemons, limes, other citrus, and citrus juices)

berries (strawberries, blueberries, raspberries)

eggs

fish (shellfish, whitefish)

peanuts (peanut butter or other products)

tomato (pizza, spaghetti sauce, catsup, and tomato by-products)

yeast (dried fruits, vinegar, mushrooms, bread, pickles, and others)

soybean (soy sauce, soy lecithin, and tofu)
carob
chocolate
colas, coffee, tea
beans
peas

Include the following foods in your diet during this period:

fresh poultry
fresh meats
vegetables (except the listed varieties)
fruits (except the listed varieties)
rice cereals
water

PHASE 2—REINTRODUCTION

After two weeks, reintroduce foods slowly, one at a time every two days. If you feel more pain when you reintroduce a food, stop the new food immediately until the symptoms clear. Use the food elimination diet under the careful supervision of a physician and/or licensed nutritionist to make sure you get adequate nutrition.

A Word of Caution: Watch Out for Additives

There is some evidence that fibromyalgia patients may feel less pain if they eliminate monosodium glutamate (MSG) and aspartame, which are found in many processed foods. You should be aware of some processed foods that contain these ingredients, even though they may be listed under other names:

- Autolyzed yeast
- Calcium caseinate
- Gelatin
- Glutamate

- Glutamic acid
- Hydrolyzed protein
- Monopotassium glutamate
- Monosodium glutamate
- Sodium caseinate
- Textured protein
- Yeast extract
- Yeast food
- Yeast nutrient

An Alkaline Dlet

The arthritis diet is an alkaline diet used by some patients for the treatment of osteoarthritis, rheumatoid arthritis, and other conditions where overacidity is thought to play a part. Naturopaths believe that arthritis is caused by the accumulation of toxic acids in the joints. These acids are thought to come naturally from the intestine, and from a failure of the body's metabolism to detoxify them when in excess in the diet. Although dietary changes, such as following a vegetarian diet, have proven to be helpful for patients with rheumatoid arthritis, studies are still inconclusive for those with fibromyalgia.

A Fibromyalgia Diet

Some people with fibromyalgia find that highly acidic foods, such as citrus products, foods in the nightshade family (tomato products, potatoes, eggplant, peppers, tobacco), red meat, cow's milk products, brown and white wheat flour products, sugar-containing foods, coffee, chocolate, and honey, seem to trigger more muscle pain. Eliminating foods to reduce pain is strictly personal and must be done on a case-by-case basis.

If you do try a food-restrictive diet, such as the one offered here, be sure to check with your physician or nutritionist about nutrient supplements that you may need.

AN ALKALINE DIET FOR ARTHRITIS

FOODS TO AVOID	FOODS TO EAT
Red meat	Whitefish, lentils, peas, chicken, eggs (no more than 4 per week)
Cow's milk, cheese, and yogurt	Goat's milk and cheese, soy milk
Brown, white, wheat flour	Oats, brown rice, corn, buckwheat, millet, 100% rye crispbread
Citrus fruit	Tomatoes (no more than twice a week), all other fruit, all vegetables
Dry roasted nuts	All other nuts, especially hazelnuts, almonds, cashews, and walnuts
Sugar and foods containing sugar, syrup, honey	Sugarcane, molasses, dried fruit, sugar-free products
Coffee, decaf coffee, cocoa, tea, alcohol	Grain coffees, herbal teas, unsweetened fruit juices, vegetable juices
Salt, pepper, vinegar	Ruthmol salt, cubes of vegetarian stock
Butter and margarine	Vegetable oil
Chocolate	Carob

Remember: Calories Still Count

Comprehensive studies on fibromyalgia are beginning to connect being overweight with a lower pain threshold, meaning you feel pain at a greater intensity. Maintaining an ideal weight is most compatible with optimal health and controlling your FMS symptoms. If years of deprivation dieting to stay slim have stressed your body, causing your metabolism to slow down and making it difficult to lose weight, you owe it to yourself and your family to stop dieting and get in control of your eating habits.

No matter how many pounds you need to lose to reach a normal weight, keep in mind that calories still count. The American Dietetics Association recommends a calorie level of *no less than ten times your desired weight,* with women getting at least 1,200 calories and men getting at least 1,400 calories per day. For instance, if your goal is 140 pounds, you should eat around 1,400 calories per day. If your goal is 180 pounds, then you can follow a diet of 1,800 calories per day for weight reduction. This daily calorie allowance will not allow a quick reduction of weight, but studies show that it is better to make lifestyle changes and lose weight slowly to make the adjustment less stressful—and stress is not something you want to add to your daily life! Gradual behavior modification is more likely to be successful, especially in terms of keeping the weight under control.

Knowing that fad diets don't work for permanent weight loss, you have to make two simple changes to get to a normal, healthy weight:

1. Change your eating habits for good.
2. Continually move around more.

Now by moving around more, I don't mean walking from one room in your home to the next. A large amount of exercise is needed to burn up calories. For example, a man weighing 180 pounds who jogs at six miles per hour for one hour will burn off 756 calories. If he eats a double burger and fries at a local fast food restaurant for lunch after his run, he has taken in approximately 800 calories or more than he burned off initially. This is not the way to lose weight!

For my patients who wish to lose weight, I recommend that they accumulate at least thirty minutes of low- to moderate-intensity physical activity every day of the week or enough to burn about 200 calories (equal to a brisk two-mile walk). Not only will exercise burn fat, it will also lower your cholesterol level, build muscle and bone, and improve your mental health. Interestingly, if you didn't change what you ate yet burned an additional 200 calories a day, you would lose about 20 pounds in one year.

Remember, as you aim to reduce FMS symptoms, work on losing a few pounds by counting calories; it is essential in controlling intake of excessive calories and managing a normal weight. Ask your doctor or a certified nutritionist for a calorie-counting guide, and keep an accurate assessment of the foods you eat each day, along with the portion size. If you go over your calorie limit, cut back the next day or increase your exercise.

COMMON WAYS TO BURN 200 CALORIES A DAY*

ACTIVITY	MINUTES TO BURN 200 CALORIES
aerobics (high/low impact)	20
bicycling (12 mph)	22
cleaning	54
cooking	72
dancing	30
dusting	82
food shopping	60
jogging (5 mph)	26
making beds	82
mowing lawn (power)	58
playing tag with kids	30
stair climbing	20
stationary cycling (10 mph)	32
tennis (doubles)	52
typing	78
vacuuming	34
walking (3 mph)	54
walking (4 mph)	36

*Based on a 130-pound woman.

washing car	40
weeding garden	38
weight training	40

In short, good nutrition can help you take an active role in your health and healing. Although there are no guarantees that the foods you eat will heal your fibromyalgia, we do know that good nutrition offers tremendous benefits of increased energy and boosts your immune system to the point where it can cope with the symptoms and fight off other serious illnesses.

10

STEP 7:
SEEK SUPPORT

Living with fibromyalgia is not easy. You may often feel that no one understands the pain, fatigue, and stress that you feel twenty-four hours a day, month after month, year after year. If prolonged, these overwhelming feelings of isolation can become a stumbling block in your quest for wellness, resulting in increased stress, anxiety, and difficulty obtaining restful sleep, not to mention difficulty in keeping healthy relationships.

It does not have to be this way. You can and must seek support to keep fibromyalgia symptoms under control and to feel whole. Whether your main support comes from your physician, a personal friend, a support group of fibromyalgia patients, or even strangers on the Internet, there are caring contacts available—if you seek them.

See an Arthritis Specialist, If Needed

Because fibromyalgia is a rheumatic disease like arthritis, obtaining proper help begins with a specific and accurate diagnosis from a physician who understands the syndrome. I suggest that you start with your primary physician, and then, if needed, seek confirmation from a board-certified rheumatologist, a specialist who diagnoses and treats fibromyalgia daily.

Beyond the initial diagnosis are a host of professionals, from physical therapists and psychologists to sleep disorder specialists and dietitians, who can help you implement the 7-Step Treatment Program as defined in this book.

Increase Your Social Support

Social support is defined as the sum of all the relationships that make you feel as if you matter to the people who matter to you. Studies have verified that a strong group of family members and close friends or a support system (doctors, nurses, other health-care professionals) can help in coping with a chronic illness such as fibromyalgia. In some cases, having this social strength has been associated with people's greater adherence to medical regimens and use of health services.

Studies now conclude that people with strong social support tend to fare better in every life situation, particularly when confronted with a chronic illness like fibromyalgia. While you may have no control over your illness, having a strong group of supportive family members and friends is something you can control. You can select the people who give you social support—even when you cannot choose events that occur in your life.

Stanford researcher Dr. David Spiegel, an expert in behavioral medicine, is widely recognized for his studies of breast cancer patients. Through years of research, Spiegel discovered that patients with advanced breast cancer that participated in weekly group therapy and social support sessions had significantly greater survival times than patients who did not participate in such groups. From his work, Spiegel concluded that social support might be a means by which to buffer the effects of stress. I believe this applies to those with any chronic illness including fibromyalgia.

Consider a Fibromyalgia Support Group

Everyone needs someone to talk to. It may be a good idea to branch out and join a fibromyalgia support group as you experience give-and-take with other sufferers.

Support is necessary for coping with any chronic illness. A support group is geared toward the unique needs of its members and is especially important for fibromyalgia patients. Although support groups are not psychotherapy groups, they do provide patients with a safe and accepting place to vent their frustrations, share their situations, and receive comfort and encouragement from one another. In many such groups, the latest methods of treatment are discussed and members give coping suggestions that you may not be aware of. Assurance is given that someone else knows what you are going through, as people share their struggles in living with this mysterious syndrome. This camaraderie is necessary in order to help you revamp your thought processes. After joining such a group, you may realize that the best experts on a disease are often those who live with it daily, although you should always check with your physician before taking a new remedy.

Fibromyalgia support groups are active around the world. Call the Fibromyalgia Association or the Arthritis Foundation (see Resources, page 287) for more information on support groups in your area. You may also check with your physician or local hospitals to see if such groups are registered. If you cannot find a group, the Fibromyalgia Association or Arthritis Foundation can provide you with information on how to start one yourself.

Try Internet Support Groups

If you would prefer not to join a group, you can find support in the privacy of your home or office on the Internet. You can exchange E-mail with those in foreign countries, who may, in turn, suggest excellent remedies that may not be popular in the United States. When going on-line, check out the World Wide

Web for the latest information on fibromyalgia, along with current periodicals and studies on the disease.

On the World Wide Web, you can visit the USA Fibrositis Association home page and the Fibromyalgia news group, among many.

Seek Support from Loved Ones

"I know she is sick, but to be honest, she looks very healthy to me." Tom came to see me about his wife, Claire, to try to find more information on fibromyalgia.

"My boss thinks I'm lazy," Ellen cried during a recent appointment after living with this disease for three years. "I cannot convince him that even though I look normal on the outside, I'm far from being normal on the inside."

Fibromyalgia's reach extends beyond the patient and can affect the entire family. Especially with such a chronic pain-related disease, personal support is necessary, whether from your spouse, family, friends, or coworkers.

It is important to educate your friends and loved ones about your disease, sensitizing them to the symptoms that may come and go but can be immobilizing at times. I have found that not only should the patient be told how to treat this disease, but it is helpful to explain the protocol for treatment to those close to the patient.

Family members can have the best of intentions, but without specific guidance, they sometimes make things worse. Family meetings with a licensed mental health counselor are another way of helping everyone deal with the stress of your disease and may be necessary if lifestyle changes have to be made to accommodate your problems.

Consider a Comprehensive Pain Clinic

If you are still having great pain after months of using the suggested 7-Step Treatment Program in this book, it may be necessary to seek additional support from a comprehensive pain clinic.

Most pain clinics use a multidisciplinary approach to treatment, including medical treatment, physical therapy, and psychological approaches to pain control. As you have learned by reading this book, each of these areas is important and complements the others.

Health care specialists at comprehensive pain clinics usually see more severe cases of deep muscle pain since, by the time of admission, most patients have tried a myriad of other treatments. Even with these more difficult cases, many comprehensive pain clinics across the nation are finding that patients are twice as likely to return to work after comprehensive pain treatment than after other treatments alone. In fact, 40 to 60 percent of the patients with chronic pain treated in comprehensive clinics return to work and report having less pain and improved activity. Considering that these patients had not responded to most other treatments, the figures are encouraging.

HOW TO CHOOSE A PAIN UNIT

The American Chronic Pain Association recommends considering the following guidelines prior to selecting a pain unit. You can contact this organization at P.O. Box 850, Rocklin, CA 95677 or call (916) 632-0922. Your personal physician can refer you to a unit, but many programs accept self-referral.

1. Make sure you locate a legitimate program. Facilities that offer pain management should include several specific components, listed below.
   • The Commission on Accreditation of Rehabilitation Facilities (CARF) (telephone: [800] 444-8991) can provide you with a listing of accredited pain programs in your area

(your health insurance may require that the unit be CARF-accredited in order for you to receive reimbursement).

• You can also contact the American Pain Society, a group of health care providers, at (708) 966-5595, for additional information about pain units in your area.

2. Choose a good program that is convenient for you and your family.

• Many pain-management programs do not offer outpatient care. Choosing a program close to your home will enable you to commute to the program each day.

3. Learn something about the people who run the program.

• Try to meet several of the staff members to get a sense of the people you will be dealing with while on the unit.

• The program should have a complete medical staff trained in pain-management techniques including:

√ Physician (may be a specialist from several different areas but should have expertise in pain management)

√ Registered nurse

√ Psychiatrist or psychologist

√ Physical therapist

√ Occupational therapist

√ Biofeedback therapist

√ Family counselor

√ Vocational counselor

√ Personnel trained in pain-management intervention

4. Make sure the program includes most of the following features:

Biofeedback training

Counseling

Family counseling

TENS (Transcutaneous Electrical Nerve Stimulation) units

Group therapy

Occupational therapy

Assertiveness training

Regional anesthesia (nerve blocks)

Physical therapy (exercise and body mechanics training, not massage, whirlpool, etc.)

Relaxation training and stress management

Educational program covering medications and other aspects of pain and its management

Aftercare (follow-up support once you have left the unit)

5. Be sure your family can be involved in your care.

- Family members should be required to be involved in your treatment.
- If you choose an out-of-town unit, find out if your family can be involved in your care.
- The program should provide special educational sessions for family members.
- Joint counseling for you and your family should also be available.

6. Also consider these additional factors:

- What services will your insurance company reimburse, and what will you be expected to cover?
- What is the unit's physical setup (is it in a patient care area or in an area by itself)?
- Is the program inpatient or outpatient (when going through medication detoxification, inpatient care is recommended)?
- Do you understand what will be required of you during your stay (length of time you will be on unit, responsibility to take care of personal needs, etc.)?
- Does the unit provide any type of job retraining?
- Make sure that, before accepting you, the unit reviews your previous medical records and gives you a complete physical evaluation to be sure you can participate in the program.
- Obtain copies of your recent medical records to prevent duplicate testing.

- Try to talk with both present and past program participants to get their feedback about their stay on the unit.

Consider the expense before you go to a pain clinic. It should be the last resort with fibromyalgia and considered only if all other methods of treatment fail.

Seeking Support with a Therapist

The fibromyalgia patient deals with pain on a daily basis and the reason for the pain is genuine—there is something wrong in the body. For most people, the last thing you want to hear is, "I think it might be a good idea for you to speak with someone about the depression and stress you have." You may conclude that the "someone" is either a psychiatrist, psychologist, or counselor of some type—a "shrink." You may be offended by the implication that the disease is "in your head." You may even become suspicious that this person does not believe that you are really feeling the pain and fatigue that you describe.

It is a fact that all people with pain, whether from fibromyalgia or other diseases, have stress, which in turn makes it more difficult to handle everyday issues, much less crisis situations that may arise. One fibromyalgia patient, Sandra, who had severe muscle pain in her shoulders, described her personality as "Dr. Jekyll and Mr. Hyde."

"Depending on whether I've slept well or not, my personality changes with the wind. I warn family and friends not to take offense when I come across irritable or irrational," she said.

Psychological counseling can help you develop appropriate and workable coping strategies to deal with the issues that affect you. It is an accepted treatment for anyone—not just people who have psychological problems or diseases.

If you do seek psychological intervention, not only will you learn new coping methods, but you will also obtain the much-needed support of a professional who understands your feelings and emotions. It is most helpful if your therapist is trained in the area of pain management and/or fibromyalgia.

You may select a one-on-one session with a therapist. These sessions may include specific help with alleviating depression, anxiety, or stress, along with many other problem areas addressed more specifically in the following section. Other sessions may include a meeting with family members or a group session, such as a support group.

Information Organizations and Support Groups

There is also support available from numerous organizations across the nation. These groups can provide you with brochures on fibromyalgia and related problems and assist you with finding a physician, support group, or pain clinic, if needed. See Resources, on pages 285 to 291.

The pressures of living with a chronic disease can overwhelm you, but it does not have to be this way, as support is available. Ask your doctor to recommend professional help and resources, including psychologists, support groups, or other patients who have fibromyalgia and want to help others. Send away for pamphlets and brochures from national organizations listed in the Resources section of this book, or go on-line and plug into a support group on the Internet.

Support from others can help you realize that you are not alone in dealing with fibromyalgia and can give new confidence as you learn to handle the daily challenges in a reasonable manner.

11

QUESTIONS PATIENTS ASK ABOUT FIBROMYALGIA

I believe that learning from others who have fibromyalgia is an excellent way to gain control over the disease's long-lasting symptoms. The following commonly asked questions will reinforce your understanding of the disease and the practical and medical responses for coping that you've learned from this book.

Q. I try to eat a varied diet but wonder if I might also need vitamins. Which are recommended?

A. Although your doctor or a certified nutritionist would be the best person to guide you, you may start with the following:

Vitamin C: 250 to 1,000 mg daily
Vitamin E: 200 to 400 IU daily
Multivitamin/mineral: 100 percent of the RDA for most vitamins and minerals
Folic acid: 400 IU daily (usually contained in multivitamin/mineral tablet)
Calcium supplement: 1,000 to 1,500 mg daily
Add other nutritional supplements as suggested by your health care professional.

Q. I was a cross-country runner in college, but in my senior year I was in an automobile accident. Since that time four years ago, I have ached all over from deep muscle pain. My doctor mentioned that I might have fibromyalgia. Do you think it was caused by the accident?

A. The chances are great that it could be related. Researchers in Israel studied people who had undergone severe stress such as military combat situations, severe auto accidents, work accidents, or terrorist incidents. They found that 21 percent of these patients also had fibromyalgia. They concluded that there may be a possible association between stress and pain, such as in fibromyalgia.

Q. I have many symptoms that are similar to those in fibromyalgia, yet my doctor insists that I have chronic fatigue syndrome. How are these ailments different?

A. Chronic fatigue syndrome (CFS) has fatigue that has been present for six months or more, which is often severe enough to cause a patient to go to bed, not to leave the home, or to be unable to work. The symptoms may begin after an illness that seems like a virus or flu, but most patients feel that it started suddenly. Problems sleeping, concentrating, and remembering recent events are common.

Like fibromyalgia, pain and stiffness in the joints and muscles are common. Headaches and fatigue after exercise are also common. Sleep is usually a problem, and many patients find sleep is not restful. Just as with FMS, there are no specific tests available to tell the diagnosis of chronic fatigue syndrome. Your doctor must make the diagnosis based on evaluation of all of your signs and symptoms. The treatment of chronic fatigue syndrome is similar to that of fibromyalgia.

Q. Why does my fibromyalgia seem to act up when the weather gets cold or very humid? My husband says I am imagining this, but I know it's true.

A. The effect of changes in weather is real. Those with arthritis or any type of chronic pain will notice higher levels of aches and pains during inclement weather or when weather fronts pass their locale. In fact, about 60 to 70 percent of patients notice changes in their pain with weather changes.

Fibromyalgia is one of the types of arthritis most sensitive to weather changes. Some researchers even include this as a characteristic part of fibromyalgia. The most common weather changes that can affect pain control are brometric pressure, humidity, and temperature. Most patients find that their pain is worse when these weather conditions change, whether the conditions are good or bad. Some patients feel better with cold and rainy weather with low barometric pressure, whereas others feel worse under the same conditions. Still others may not notice any difference with the weather. Some weather reports now include "pain forecasts" for areas that are more likely to notice changes in arthritis pain and stiffness.

Try the following suggestions when the weather changes and you expect to be affected:

- Treat it like a flare-up of fibromyalgia, and even before it happens, be sure you're doing twice-daily moist heat (shower, bath, whirlpool, hot tub).
- Continue to exercise in the shower or immediately after, gradually increasing toward your goal of twenty repetitions of each exercise, twice daily.
- Keep up your walking or bicycling, working up to twenty to thirty minutes each day.
- Continue your medications that have proven to be effective in the past.
- Continue your complementary/alternative treatment program.

Q. How do you know if a new medication or treatment will really work for FMS? I've heard about some miracle cures lately and would love to try one—if I knew they'd work.

A. Although many common health problems like FMS have no cure, there will always be treatments offered by well-meaning

ربط

family members and friends who want you to have relief of pain and tiredness. Some people will tell you how a new treatment worked for them. These "personal testimonials" might seem appealing. After all, who would want to miss the chance for relief, even if it may not be proven or approved by the FDA?

Nonetheless, the nagging question remains: How can you get the benefit of new treatments for FMS but avoid the bad ones? What if your doctor is needlessly avoiding a good treatment?

You can best protect yourself from wasting both time and money by becoming an expert. Learn about FMS by getting information from your doctor, the library, and the Internet. The information available on the Internet is almost unlimited and can give you a good idea of the current standard and nonstandard or complementary treatments. You can find where to go to get the best available diagnosis and treatment for your FMS. Each source can lead you to other ways to learn more about each treatment. The more you know, the better you will understand FMS, and the better you'll be at helping your doctor decide your own best plan to get the best relief of pain.

A few questions may help you sort out treatments that are more legitimate and safe. Ask:

What are the side effects?
Is it safe for long-term treatment?
Was it tested in trials approved by the FDA?
What has happened to similar treatments over the years?

Even if you aren't sure about a treatment for FMS, if it is harmless and doesn't delay a proper diagnosis and known treatment, it's okay to try it. Many ointments, rubs, and creams are good examples. A copper bracelet for arthritis doesn't hurt and some feel better just by wearing one. But in some areas, remedies such as rattlesnake meat in capsules was found to cause severe illness or death.

Most of our FMS patients have tried one or more types of complementary treatments. Just remember to continue with the treatment methods we know will help, such as moist heat and exercise, while you check out the safe nonstandard treatments. Take advantage of new ideas but avoid those that may cause more harm than good.

Q. I've had fibromyalgia since my early twenties. I'm planning to get pregnant this year and wondered if this will worsen my pain and fatigue.

A. It's good that you are thinking ahead, trying to understand what your body may go through with a change such as pregnancy. In other types of arthritis, such as rheumatoid arthritis, patients often have improvement in pain and stiffness during pregnancy. Unfortunately, most studies have revealed a worsening of the symptoms of fibromyalgia. In fact, most patients feel worse for the first three months after pregnancy, with some studies revealing as many as 80 percent of women having increased symptoms.

Since stress, both physical and emotional, is known to aggravate fibromyalgia, it is not surprising that symptoms can be worse during and after pregnancy. Pregnancy and delivery are high-stress times, both physically and emotionally, with large changes in the levels of estrogen, progesterone, and other hormones. Since the time after a pregnancy can be difficult for mothers even without the added pain of fibromyalgia, it is important to be aware of the possible increase in pain that can occur then, too.

The good news is that there are some steps that can be taken to help reduce stress during and after pregnancy. Make sure you get regular rest periods, two or three times each day for twenty to thirty minutes each time. This will help you improve the quality of the rest of the day and evening. Be sure to use moist heat twice daily (a warm shower or bath, along with gentle stretching exercises). While pregnant, do not use a whirlpool spa or hot water in your bath, as it could endanger the fetus.

Talk with your doctor about the type and use of medications to control pain and stiffness just as you would at other times during the treatment of fibromyalgia. You might try some of the alternative therapies outlined in chapter 7. A gentle massage, the relaxation response, and music therapy are all easy ways to de-stress and can be done during pregnancy. A word of caution: Be sure to check with your doctor before taking any of the herbs listed in chapter 7. And after the pregnancy, if you breast feed, be sure you check with your doctor before you take any medications.

Q. I was diagnosed with fibromyalgia about three years ago. This past week my doctor told me I also have TMJ and must get a dental appliance to wear during sleep. What is TMJ and what can I do to ease the pain in my jaw and ear?

A. TMJ syndrome is very common in women, in fact, from 80 to 95 percent of the cases affect women. It can start as early as the teenage years or in the twenties. Pain is felt in the muscles used for chewing, with areas of localized tenderness and sensations of popping or clicking. It may be hard to completely open the jaw, due to pain when chewing. Many patients complain of clicking sensations, even though they are also common in otherwise healthy people. Many experts think clicking sensations alone are not a sign of serious disease.

To relieve symptoms of TMJ pain, avoid chewy food, including gum and sticky candy, and eat soft foods for several days. Also, take nonsteroid anti-inflammatory medications (NSAIDs) or COX-2 medications (see page 78) to ease the swelling and pain. While these medications do not cure TMJ, they reduce the pain so you can start to exercise the joint. A warm moist towel applied to the jaw for a few minutes several times each day can also work wonders in alleviating pain and stiffness. Another choice is an ice pack placed over the TMJ area for a few minutes, being careful to place the ice in a towel and not directly on the skin.

It's also important to exercise the jaw joint and surrounding muscles, even though it may seem difficult at first. Exercises can help to make your muscles stronger and more flexible, which gives the joints more support. Ask your doctor or dentist to show you some simple isometric jaw exercises you can do at home to strengthen the muscles around the jaw.

Your dentist plays a key role in making sure no other problem is causing the jaw pain. Some causes of jaw pain are related to the teeth and might need antibiotics for infection or a procedure to drain an infected root. A custom-fitted splint (biteplate, nightguard) worn at night may reduce pain as it helps to end key causes of TMJ syndrome, such as bruxism (grinding of the teeth) and clenching of the jaw. Medications, as discussed on page 76, such as amitriptyline and imipramine may give relief. In some cases, injections or arthroscopic surgery may be needed, depending on the problem.

Talk to your doctor about a psychological evaluation for stress management as high stress can also result in chronic muscle tension. Some studies show that more than 85 percent of all TMJ cases are caused by muscle tension in the jaw, face, neck, and shoulders. Identifying your stress triggers and controlling your stress response may help to alleviate this common cause of facial pain.

Q. Is it normal for my symptoms to flare up the week before my menstrual period? I am achy and exhausted, and I toss and turn at night for about five days before my period. What can I do to relieve this?

A. It is very common to have aggravation of symptoms during the week before your menstrual period starts. Knowing that this is true, you can take "preventive" measures to avoid worsening of the symptoms.

Stay with your twice-daily moist heat, exercise, and stretch each day, and continue with the medications your doctor has prescribed. Read pages 233 to 235 in chapter 9 and follow the suggestions for dietary control to ease PMS symptoms. Perhaps more important, watch your schedule. Try to avoid a high-stress week with too many commitments. Staying home during the evenings and relaxing the week prior to your period may help you to unwind and sleep more soundly. Try one of the calming herbs such as chamomile (chapter 7) in a warm tea before bedtime, and see if this may give relief.

Q. I have lived with fibromyalgia symptoms for six years, and my doctor recently diagnosed it as a specific disease. She sent me to a fibromyalgia support group in our city, and thirty-two of the thirty-eight members were women around my age (age forty-nine). Does this mean that fibromyalgia is a middle-aged woman's disease?

A. It is really common to be bothered by the feelings of fibromyalgia for years before an exact diagnosis is made. Once the diagnosis is made, however, the picture becomes clear. Only then can proper treatment begin.

Support groups for fibromyalgia are a great source of information. This is a good way to keep up with the latest research and treatments available. Dealing with fibromyalgia alone can be discouraging; it helps to talk openly with others who have dealt with the problem successfully. Also, you may be able to help others.

Yes, it is a fact that most fibromyalgia patients are women, but it can happen to men. About 90 percent of patients (nine in ten) are women, commonly in the middle years of life.

Q. I keep hearing that this is a woman's disease, yet I am a six-foot-two male who was recently diagnosed with fibromyalgia. Could there be a hormonal problem that is causing this to happen to my body? If so, what treatment would be effective?

A. Although it is true that the vast majority of cases of fibromyalgia happen in women, it is also true that men suffer from this disease as well. The specific causes are not known. In our clinic, we do see fibromyalgia in men at times and some of them have had a severe injury to the back, such as a ruptured disc in the lumbar spine, months or even years before.

There is no evidence that hormones play a role in fibromyalgia in men. The treatment is the same for both men and women, and by staying on my 7-Step Treatment Program, you should obtain relief.

Q. I was diagnosed with fibromyalgia after having great pain stemming from a hysterectomy. I had pain when I awoke, and then more pain throughout the day. Then it seemed as if my bladder completely shut down. I was rushed to the emergency room for a catheterization and was told it was part of fibromyalgia. Have you ever heard of this happening?

A. Fibromyalgia can begin after a very stressful situation, an injury, or a serious illness. Some women have found that it began after a hysterectomy. Remember, the causes are just not known. Many problems other than pain and stiffness can result, such as abdominal pain, bloating, constipation and diarrhea, and irritable bowel syndrome (IBS).

Also, as discussed on page 31, urinary frequency, the urge to urinate, and pain on urination can come with fibromyalgia. There is no special treatment other than the treatment of the disease itself and certain medicines that can help the bladder control.

Talk to your doctor to be sure you have the best combination of medicines to control the symptoms of this disease.

Q. My family practitioner is treating me for fibromyalgia, but I feel that I need a specialist. What type of doctor would you recommend for this disease? Are there certain tests I will need?

A. See your family doctor first, but if your fibromyalgia is not improved after a reasonable amount of time (say a few months), then yes, it is a good idea to ask for an opinion from a rheumatologist. Rheumatologists deal with arthritis and related diseases. They treat many patients with fibromyalgia. This specialist will review your diagnosis and coordinate the plan for treatment.

The diagnosis of fibromyalgia is still made from an examination and talking with the patient. A few blood tests and X rays will help to eliminate other types of arthritis. This is important to be sure that no other specific treatments will be needed. If the rheumatologist agrees with the diagnosis of fibromyalgia, a plan for treatment can be made.

Q. After a lengthy bout with the flu, my seventeen-year-old daughter was diagnosed with fibromyalgia. Is this common?

A. Fibromyalgia does happen in teenagers. Although uncommon, it causes the same pain, stiffness, and fatigue that adults experience. It usually improves slowly over time. The course of treatment may be helped by a regular program of moist heat, exercises, and medication, as discussed in chapter 4. Just as in adults, fibromyalgia in teenagers seems to follow a severe injury or illness, but the exact reason why is not known.

Q. Does taking estrogen have anything to do with fibromyalgia? After a complete hysterectomy at age thirty-five, my doctor put me on estrogen replacement. Within one year, I developed horrible muscle pain and fatigue that would not end, even with bed rest. Was it the estrogen? If so, what should I do?

A. There is no good evidence that the hysterectomy or the estrogen treatment is the cause of fibromyalgia, although fibromyalgia does occur in some women after a hysterectomy. The surgery as well as the estrogen treatment are common events in many women. Unless your doctor advises otherwise, you can continue your estrogen treatment without fear of aggravating your fibromyalgia.

However, in some patients with fibromyalgia, there does seem to be a major illness, injury, or emotional stress just before the start of their symptoms. It is not known how these events seem to trigger fibromyalgia. Perhaps future research will bring this answer to light.

Q. Fibromyalgia has taken over my life and is taking over my family's life as well. Is there a cure for this, or will it continue to cause pain forever? Growing older with all this pain does not seem appealing. What does research show for the future?

A. The chronic pain and fatigue can certainly take over your life. It can cause avoidance of your usual activities, less exercise, more pain, and a vicious cycle of further withdrawal, which can lead to depression. The chronic pain of fibromyalgia can change your personality, making it difficult to get along with those you love.

Although there is no cure and no prediction about how long the disease will take to run its course, it's important that your family shares in your disease. When you are tired, stressed, and in pain, it affects how your family feels and acts.

A big problem in fibromyalgia is that the patient does not appear to be sick. There are few outward signs of pain. The frustration from your inability to keep up with your activities shows to others in the way you act. It is a good idea to see a clinical psychologist or psychiatrist for tips on stress management. This professional can be invaluable in helping you deal with the stress of chronic pain.

Right now, there is no cure for fibromyalgia in sight, but good treatment is available and will work if you stick to the 7-Step Program. Most patients eventually improve with treatment. Your goals might be to have a reasonable relief of the pain and tiredness so that you can get around and do the things you need to do each day.

Q. I am the mother of three daughters and was recently diagnosed with fibromyalgia. Does this mean that my daughters will also be subject to this disease? Are there prevention methods?

A. If you have the diagnosis of fibromyalgia, it does not mean that your daughters are also destined to be sufferers. The causes of fibromyalgia are unknown. Since there are no known ways to prevent fibromyalgia, I suggest that you simply keep up a good exercise program, including maintaining your cardiovascular fitness, and encourage your daughters to do the same. There is some evidence that an ongoing exercise program, including good conditioning, may make a person more resistant to fibromyalgia.

Q. I started the daily exercise program, but on some days just getting out of bed is a chore. Then, after I exercise, I ache even more. Should I push myself even when the pain and fatigue are unbearable?

A. Most patients with fibromyalgia feel stiff on awakening in the morning. It may even take an hour or more to loosen up. These feelings are very much a part of the disease. Usually, when there is relief of other symptoms with treatment, there is also improvement in the morning stiffness.

It is also typical to have worsening of the aching and pain after exercise. This is a big problem, since it can make patients avoid exercise, an important healing component of the 7-Step Treatment Program. In our clinic, we suggest that patients do their best to keep up the regular exercise program, on good and bad days.

Aerobic exercise, such as an exercise class, walking, bicycling, or swimming, should be continued daily, if possible. On bad days, you might do a little less, but try not to stop completely. Gradually increase back to your old level as soon as you feel less pain.

Remember, on days when you feel better, you may be tempted to totally skip exercise. Don't let this happen!

Regular exercise can help you have more good days in the future.

Q. I started NSAIDs for the muscle aches of fibromyalgia, but they did little for the pain. Without purchasing a host of medications, is there a way to tell which medication will help most?

A. NSAIDs (nonsteroidal anti-inflammatory drugs) may not help at all in fibromyalgia. This is because there is little inflammation present in the tissues, if fibromyalgia is the only problem. But these medications may also be used as pain relievers, so you may try them for that reason.

There are more than twenty NSAIDs available on the market. Most people find one that works without side effects, but it may be necessary to try a number of different types to find the one that is best. Ask your doctor to make a suggestion. In our clinic we try to provide our patients with manufacturer samples. When a patient finds a sample medication that works effectively, then the medication can be purchased.

If you notice any new problems, such as nausea, then check with your doctor to see if you should continue using this NSAID.

Q. My doctor told me that my constant pain and fatigue were caused by fibromyalgia, even though my lab tests were normal. How can she be sure that this is fibromyalgia and not some other disease?

A. There are no specific blood tests or other tests that can definitely make the diagnosis of fibromyalgia, but these tests can help rule out certain diseases. The diagnosis is made by the symptoms you express to your doctor: the widespread pain, the trigger points, typical fatigue, depression, and other problems, as discussed in chapter 3. Some of the most common problems that may also be present with fibromyalgia include osteoarthritis, rheumatoid arthritis, and other types of arthritis or thyroid disease. Each of these problems has specific symptoms and tests for diagnosis.

Q. Can't I speed up the course of fibromyalgia? I've had this disease for seven years and see no end in sight.

A. Fibromyalgia can last for years, but there are definite steps you can take to control the symptoms. There is no cure at this time, but the program of moist heat, exercises, medication, and other measures can make the pain tolerable. If you can control your pain and do most of your usual activities, you can win against fibromyalgia.

Many researchers have found that after a few years, the limitations from fibromyalgia are fewer. Many people still have some pain but not the severe and widespread pain and fatigue that was present in earlier years. One study found 24 percent of patients developed excellent control of their symptoms. About 50 percent of patients in the same study experienced more frequent pain-free periods. You can speed up the improvement of the disease with the 7-Step Treatment Program described in this book.

Q. What about moist heat in the treatment of fibromyalgia? I bought a Jacuzzi in hopes that this would help alleviate my constant pain.

A. I don't know of anyone who has not felt totally relaxed after spending time in a Jacuzzi or whirlpool bath. Hot baths are part of one of the oldest methods of alternative treatments for chronic pain associated with arthritis, specifically fibromyalgia. The Romans built baths to provide warm pools for treatment, and the theory behind these baths is just as useful today. The moist heat gives soothing relief to painful muscle aches and provides comfort just as in today's treatments. Many times after relaxing in a whirlpool or Jacuzzi, you are able to do your exercises easily, without as much muscle pain.

Q. Why do you keep saying to exercise when I can hardly get out of the chair? I cannot imagine starting a walking or biking program with the pain I have.

A. Many researchers find exercise to be one of the most important parts of the treatment of fibromyalgia, because it can help improve endurance and strength. Most fibromyalgia patients have not exercised regularly for some time because of the pain and are out of condition. However, in treating hundreds of patients with fibromyalgia, we have learned that those who start and continue an exercise program are much more likely to see their symptoms improve.

Usually, the most difficult part is starting the exercise program when you are stiff and in pain. Two types of exercise are helpful. One is endurance exercise, which gives good cardiovascular exercise and improves fitness. This can improve your ability to accomplish daily activities, reduce stress and anxiety, and help with depression.

How do you start endurance exercise? Simply make yourself start walking every day. Walk a short distance, one that you can easily accomplish, and gradually increase that distance. Or use an electronic treadmill indoors and slowly increase the time you spend on the machine.

The second type of exercise used to treat fibromyalgia is muscle-strengthening exercise. These simple exercises, described in chapter 5, can be done at home. Muscle-strengthening exercise achieves two goals: Stronger and more flexible muscles are less likely to become painful and stiff with daily activity; and stronger muscles are less likely to become tired and fatigued with activity.

Q. A friend of mine who also has fibromyalgia mentioned trying DMSO for pain relief. What is DMSO and how is it used? Is it safe?

A. DMSO (dimethyl sulfoxide) is sold in an impure form in some hardware stores and has been used to treat illnesses in horses for years. In humans, DMSO has been used by athletes to treat injuries to muscles and tendons. It is a liquid that is absorbed into the system when applied to the skin. Side effects include strong, garlicky breath odor and occasional skin irritation where it was applied. If DMSO is injected into a vein, it is very dangerous and can cause liver and other internal organ damage. This should never be done.

Although the U.S. Food and Drug Administration (FDA) has not approved DMSO for use in treating arthritis or bursitis, it has found that DMSO might be helpful in relieving pain caused by bursitis, acute injuries, and possibly rheumatoid arthritis. DMSO is used by some fibromyalgia patients. In my clinic, I see little use among fibromyalgia patients, but I do not object if it is used carefully and gives relief.

Q. What about usage of over-the-counter creams, liniments, and lotions for muscle pain relief with fibromyalgia? Are these harmful?

A. Creams, liniments, and lotions are widely advertised and used for the pain of arthritis and other conditions. Many types are available at your drugstore and at health food stores. They are not harmful when used properly and can be continued if you feel improvement in muscle pain.

One newer topical cream, capsaicin, sold over the counter under various brand names, such as Capsaicin or Zostrix, has been found to be quite beneficial in the few existing studies. One particular capsaicin lotion is available in a roll-on applicator and is sold as Capsin (ask your pharmacist for information on this product).

Capsaicin has an active ingredient derived from red chili peppers. When nerve endings in the body are touched by capsaicin, they produce *substance P,* a neurotransmitter that carries pain messages to the brain. Repeated applications of capsaicin results in fewer pain messages to the brain. Although this cream can cause warmth or a burning sensation, it does not cause blistering, and the burning feeling usually decreases the longer the cream is used.

Q. My friend told me about a cream that is only found at health food stores that is made from an herb. Do you know anything about this?

A. Boswellian Cream can be found at some health food stores and has been used for centuries to treat pain-related ailments. This cream is made of four triterpene acids from the herb *Boswellia serrata,* which has been found to bring temporary relief to minor aches and pains associated with arthritis.

Use this cream with caution, as it does produce mild inflammation and redness to the skin when applied, supposedly in order to achieve its healing properties. A loose bandage should be applied after the cream. Boswellian Cream is for external use only; if your skin becomes inflamed, stop its usage.

Q. I'm trying to use complementary treatments in controlling stress. Most specifically, I've started a regular program of guided imagery, along with progressive relaxation and deep breathing. How will I know if this is working?

A. Each person reacts differently, and some forms of mind-body therapy will be successful in some patients and less useful in others. The best results happen when the most effective methods for each patient are used for symptom relief. As always, everyone is different. The important factor is to choose those that work for you and launch out in a regular, daily program of relaxation. Monitor your heart rate as you do this. Does the relaxation help you feel calm and at ease? Continue to practice the technique(s) that you choose until you are able to elicit the relaxation response anytime during the day, especially during stressful moments.

Q. You keep emphasizing the importance of a "combination" treatment program. What exactly does this mean?

A. Let me answer that by using two interesting case studies. Patty epitomized the typical fibromyalgia patient. This thirty-seven-year-old mother maintained a very successful home-based business while caring for her four children. She volunteered at her church and helped teach computer at her children's school two afternoons a week. Although she never found time to exercise, Patty was able to maintain a normal weight simply from the nervous energy she burned balancing so many responsibilities . . . until she was diagnosed with fibromyalgia.

"It started with unending fatigue after getting the flu last winter," she said. "I kept thinking that if only I could get more sleep I would feel well, but the tiredness wouldn't go away. Then I began to feel achy all over, day after day. Sometimes I got a grinding sound in my neck when I moved it. My neck began to feel stiff all the time, as well as both shoulders, and when I touched my neck, it felt warm. My muscles would be so sore that it felt like I had exercised for hours the day before, but I hadn't. Even my scalp hurt."

Patty didn't have time to tolerate the interruption of fibromyalgia's symptoms in her busy life. I recommended her to a stress clinic in town, where she worked with the therapists using biofeedback, guided imagery, and the relaxation response. Her physical therapist referred her to a licensed massage therapist, and she went for weekly muscle massages. After three months of treatment, medication that helped her to achieve restful sleep, and a regular exercise program, Patty was feeling hopeful that she could live a normal life in spite of her disease.

Patty's experience illustrates what I have found to be true, that a combination treatment program can assist a patient in decreasing stress and pacing her lifestyle so that the symptoms of fibromyalgia are diminished or managed.

When forty-six-year-old Marilyn came to see me for an evaluation, she had experienced fibromyalgia symptoms for three years. "The symptoms began around the time my last son left for college," she told me. "At that time, I was very anxious and mildly depressed. My husband, Ray, was fully involved in his career and both boys were away at school. All I had to occupy my time was cleaning the house each day and waiting for Ray to come home from work."

Marilyn told of feeling stiffness and pain in her arms and hands, especially her right hand and thumb. She also had a pinching pain in her left hip, making it difficult to lift her foot to walk. Fibromyalgia also caused painful cramps and sharp, stabbing pains in her left calf. Her toes on the same side would suddenly pull under and cramp.

After an evaluation, I realized that Marilyn had many influences at work in her. Not only was she dealing with the symptoms of fibromyalgia, she was also confronted with what many call the "empty nest syndrome." But this woman did not seek pity. Instead, she sought the assistance of an excellent psychologist, who helped her learn some of the relaxation techniques described in chapter 7. She found music therapy and deep abdominal breathing especially helpful, particularly during stressful times.

Using a combination of treatment, including medication, exercise, moist heat, and the mind-body approach to healing, Marilyn was able to find relief. Choosing any one component of the treatment program alone will not give such outstanding relief. That is why I constantly encourage a total combination treatment program.

Q. I was watching a program on *20/20* in which the doctor said that FMS might be cured by surgery because it was part of the Chiari Malformation syndrome. What is your opinion on this—help or hype?

A. The report you are referring to found that some patients with fibromyalgia had an unusual situation involving the lower portion of the brain called Chiari Malformation. In that light, the clinician felt that the patients' fibromyalgia might be helped by surgery to correct the abnormality. To be quite honest, this abnormality is unusual enough that most fibromyalgia specialists do not routinely order an MRI test necessary to make the diagnosis of the malformation.

The surgery to correct Chiari Malformation syndrome is very complicated and does have risks. In addition, there is no proven guarantee that it will cure fibromyalgia. Talk to your doctor about this syndrome, but make sure you understand the benefits and risks and what to expect after surgery, if you ever consider this unproven treatment for fibromyalgia.

Q. I've had fibromyalgia for six years, and I've finally got the symptoms managed, using your 7-Step Treatment Program. Now I have a new problem! My sister is getting married, and I will be traveling from Maine to Oregon to attend the wedding. While I'm looking forward to flying and sightseeing, I know I'll spend most of the time in pain. Do you have some suggestions?

A. I see many patients with fibromyalgia who worry that they can no longer travel and enjoy new places. However, I believe that limiting travel can increase feelings of sadness and loss of control over your life. Travel is an important way to maintain independence and relationships, and increase your sense of well-being. If you will take the following simple steps now, you can make traveling with fibromyalgia much easier:

1. *Plan the details before the trip.* Ask your travel agent to book a hotel room with a valet service, so you won't have to carry your bags. Make sure your room is on the ground level to avoid having to climb stairs. Make sure the hotel has a dining room for easy access to meals.

2. *Arrange to travel at nonpeak hours.* Less traffic at the airport will help you to travel more easily. Talk to your travel agent about your accommodations to make sure you will have easy access to the plane. Request an airline escort who will meet you at baggage check-in and take

you to your gate in an electric cart. This must be done ahead of time, so make sure you ask for special assistance.

3. *Pack lightly.* Avoid overpacking by limiting the luggage you will take. I recommend that you take half as much as you normally would consider for a trip, and use the convenient laundry services at the hotel. Make sure your luggage is on wheels so you can easily pull it to the airport check-in counter.

4. *Stay on your exercise program.* Be sure to continue exercising in the weeks prior to the trip, as well as during your stay. This preparation will ensure that you are flexible and strong and will help you avoid increased pain from lack of activity.

5. *Remember your 7-Step Treatment Program.* While you are on the trip, stay on your medications and continue with the twice-daily moist heat baths to reduce pain and stiffness. If there is a spa facility at your hotel, schedule a massage, and use the Jacuzzi, if available. There is no reason why fibromyalgia should keep you homebound and limit your travel. With careful planning, you should be able to do all the activities you want with just a few modifications.

Q. I've been invited to go by train to Canada with a group of friends. The only problem is they are all healthy, and I have fibromyalgia. I don't want to miss this trip, but I also want to stay upbeat and not become a burden for the group. What can I do to ease the pain from sitting for long periods? Moreover, how do I keep up with my friends upon arrival when they want to sightsee?

A. You don't have to let fibromyalgia limit you from enjoying your friends and travel. Continue your exercise program during your trip—even on the train ride. With more time available, you can stand up and do stretches while riding on the train. Also, walk up and down the aisle of the train for five to ten minutes every hour to keep your muscles flexible and strong. Review the exercises on pages 109 to 118, and use these during your trip to stay pain-free.

It's important to pace yourself on the trip. When you arrive in Canada, don't feel you have to do everything in one day—even if your friends push themselves. Try to fit in a reasonable amount of sightseeing, but also allow for rest periods throughout the day. You might bring a few books to enjoy during this quiet time.

Continue with your moist heat and stay on your medications to keep symptoms at bay. If you find that the sightseeing is taxing, let your friends know you'll need more down time, and take in some movies or concerts. In other words, pace your schedule of activities so they match your energy level and don't exacerbate your symptoms.

Make sure your travel bags are light and easy to carry without increasing your pain. Also, take a large shoulder bag for your camera and personal items so you don't have to juggle many smaller bags when sightseeing. Some of my patients who travel frequently like the packs that hook around the waist like a belt. These packs are convenient for sightseeing, large enough to carry necessary items, and will not aggravate shoulder, neck, or back pain during your active day.

Q. My fifteen-year-old daughter was diagnosed with rheumatoid arthritis at age twelve. This past year she complained of body aches that would not resolve and had difficulty falling asleep, to the point where she was homeschooled the last six months of her sophomore year. Finally, her rheumatologist told us that she has fibromyalgia. What help is there for my child?

A. Fibromyalgia and rheumatoid arthritis can both happen at almost any age. If your rheumatologist has made a definite diagnosis of fibromyalgia along with rheumatoid arthritis, then this could open some effective treatment possibilities as most of the treatments for these two problems don't conflict. I would encourage your daughter to follow her rheumatologist's instructions. Helping one problem may give relief of pain and fatigue, which could make your daughter's overall function and ability to get around improve at this important time in her life.

Along with taking the proper medications, using the moist heat, and exercising daily, make sure your daughter is getting sound sleep at night. If she is having problems getting to sleep or maintaining sleep, then talk to her doctor about medications that may help resolve this. It's also important to understand that these major problems greatly affect your daughter's life, including her level of stress. Stress management by a clinical psychologist may be helpful to assist her in dealing with these health problems and how they impact her teen years.

Q. I feel like my doctor doesn't take me seriously when I tell him how I feel. Are there some ways to get his attention so he doesn't regard me as a female hysteric? Alternatively, should I just look for another doctor?

A. I doubt if your doctor has labeled you as a hysteric, but there are ways to be well prepared before your visit to help your doctor understand your signs and symptoms. Take time before your appointment to write down how you feel. Describe the pain, including the location, frequency, and severity. Write down how you are sleeping, and situations that affect your sleep habits. Also write down the amount of exercise you are getting now and if your pain improves or worsens with exercise. Be sure to add any questions you might have about fibromyalgia or the prescribed medications.

By providing your doctor with this organized information, he can treat the symptoms methodically and logically. In addition, you will be sure your questions are answered as you jot down the response or check them off your list. If you still feel your doctor has not heard you, then seek another opinion and find a doctor who listens and respects you as a patient and person.

Q. I just turned fifty and have had fibromyalgia for almost a decade. Now after suffering two wrist fractures over three years, my doctor wants to test me for osteoporosis. What tests will diagnosis this?

A. Because you are a fifty-year-old woman, osteoporosis—thinning of the bones—is a concern. In fact, osteoporosis is the most common cause of all fractures, with 1.5 to 2 million fractures annually, and it's the twelfth leading cause of death in the United States, resulting in more than 50,000 deaths annually.

As I explain in my book *The Osteoporosis Cure* (Avon, 1998), there are no signs or feelings of osteoporosis until a fracture occurs. If you have osteoporosis then the fractures are clues that could allow you to begin treatment and, hopefully, prevent future fractures, especially hip fracture, which is disabling.

Check the following list of risk factors for osteoporosis. While you cannot change the fact that you are over forty, a female, and have had a fracture, you can change the risk factors you can control, as given below. I believe it's a good idea to have the bone density test, which is a safe and accurate way to tell if osteoporosis is present. If you do have osteoporosis, talk to your doctor about treatment and ways to prevent future fractures.

Q. Since I was diagnosed with fibromyalgia, I miss gardening the most out of all my past activities. Are there some tips that might allow me to get my hands dirty again and enjoy my favorite hobby?

A. Many of my patients enjoy gardening, and you can, too. With a few minor modifications, I believe this activity can give you pleasure and allow you to increase exercise to ease aching muscles. Here are some suggestions:

1. Never kneel on hard surfaces. You can purchase a kneeling pad or stool at any gardening store.

Risk Factors for Osteoporosis

Risk Factors That Cannot Be Changed

- Genetic predisposition
- Race (Caucasians and Asian women are at greater risk)
- Sex and age (female over forty increases risk)
- History of fractures after age forty

Risk Factors That Can Be Changed

- Lack of regular exercise
- Smoking cigarettes
- Being underweight
- Heavy alcohol consumption
- Taking certain medications
- Low calcium in diet
- Menopause

2. Work in short sessions. If you are just returning to gardening and exercise, work for ten or fifteen minutes, and then take a break. Stand up, walk around, and stretch during this break to help ease muscle tightness.

3. Find special equipment to help make the job easier. There are newly designed gardening tools such as rakes, hoes, and shovels that can make the job easier. Make sure you have easy-to-use tools with long handles to reduce bending, so your hobby doesn't turn into drudgery.

4. Invest in a good cart or wheelbarrow. Avoid carrying heavy gardening equipment or bags by placing them in the cart or wheelbarrow and pushing them to the location.

5. Ask for help on the difficult tasks. If you suffer with neck or shoulder pain or carpal tunnel syndrome, ask for help in cutting back shrubs or bushes. If you have pain in the lower

back, then avoid bending over too much. Get help in lifting heavy items or digging holes for planting. You may want to pay for part-time help while you get your garden up to par, and then maintain it each day once it's established.

Q. Should I request a second opinion if my fibromyalgia symptoms do not get better after a reasonable time?

A. Yes. After a period of six to eight weeks, you should discuss your failure to progress with your doctor and discuss alternatives to the current treatment program. It is very important to communicate with your doctor and not just assume that your failure to progress is known by your doctor. Most doctors welcome a second opinion in difficult cases and will suggest the names of other doctors who might be able to help. Be sure to clear any second opinions with the insurance company paying the bills. This is very important if your bills are being paid under a restrictive HMO system.

Q. My doctor has prescribed moist heat whirlpool baths twice daily using a Jacuzzi. What should I do if my insurance company refuses to pay for this therapy?

A. Insurance plans are written to be general rather than specific. Your treatment plan may be outside the norm, resulting in the denial of benefits. If this happens, you should look at your plan booklet and find out what you should do to appeal the denial of benefits. Be sure to follow all the procedural steps in a timely manner. You should ask your doctor to write a letter to the person or committee handling your appeal explaining why the therapy and Jacuzzi are needed. At the hearing, present all the reasons for continued treatment or for the purchase of equipment. If your appeal is denied, you can seek the advice of an attorney.

Q. If the insurance company that is paying my medical bills or wage loss schedules me for a physical examination by a doctor of its choice, do I have to attend?

A. Yes. All insurance policies that provide coverage for the payment of medical bills or wage loss have provisions for "independent medical examinations." The stated reason for such examinations is to make sure your treatment is reasonable and necessary, or to make sure you are still unable to go back to work.

Many times the examinations are requested by the insurance company to establish a legal basis to suspend your benefits. The suspension is based on the examining doctor's opinion that the treatment you are receiving is not reasonable or necessary, and that you no longer need to be out of work. Since the examining doctor is paid by the insurance company, a bias in the insurance company's favor could be present.

You should advise your treating doctor of the examination and request that copies of your records and test results be sent to the examining doctor before the day of the exam so that the examining doctor will have an opportunity to review the records before coming to a conclusion regarding your case. You might also want to see your doctor on the same day as the exam so your doctor will know how you were doing before the exam. You'll be required to gather up all of your X rays and scans and take them with you to the exam.

If your benefits are suspended because of the exam, you should immediately seek the advice of an attorney. If you contest the suspension, you have a good chance of having the suspension reversed. You should keep your treating doctor advised of all the details respecting the suspension since it may be due to a lack of information on the part of the examining doctor, and your treating doctor can clear up the confusion. Any treatment received after the suspension must be paid for by you. If your attorney is subsequently successful in getting the suspension reversed, you will be reimbursed for the medical bills you paid.

Q. If I seek the advice of an attorney, what should I expect to pay and how is the payment handled?

A. State and federal laws generally provide for the recovery of an attorney's fee if a person is successful in a suit to get an insurance company to pay benefits that should have been paid voluntarily. Many attorneys are willing to handle such claims on a contingency/hourly rate basis. In other words, you would agree to pay an hourly rate, but only if the case is successful. In that event, the insurance company would pay your attorney the hourly rate fee. If your case were not successful, then you would pay nothing except for the out-of-pocket expenses incurred by your attorney in the handling of your case.

Your attorney will want to investigate your case very carefully before accepting such a fee agreement since no fee would be earned if the case is unsuccessful. You would be responsible to fully disclose all the relevant facts concerning your injury as well as any prior injuries to the same part of your body. In most all cases, you should be able to get an attorney to review your case free or for a nominal consultation charge. You would need to bring to the consultation conference a plan booklet and all correspondence related to the case. You would also need to provide your attorney with a copy of your medical records.

Q. I saw four doctors this past year and finally was diagnosed with fibromyalgia a few weeks ago. The problem is the bills are now due, and they are overwhelming—physicians, X rays, medications, and therapy. How do I know if my insurance company will pay for these?

A. Medical treatment for fibromyalgia syndrome takes time and can involve medication, physical therapy, and expensive testing. Treatment is generally covered by insurance, but the type of insurance available may vary depending on where and how your injury occurred. On-the-job injuries are generally covered by workers' compensation insurance. Injuries sustained in auto accidents are covered by a combination of auto no-fault insurance and group health insurance. Sports

injuries and injuries incurred around the house are generally only covered by group health insurance.

Many times your physician will file the forms for all services provided, but sometimes you will have to file your claim
to receive reimbursement. The process of medical claims
can be confusing and stressful. If the claim is not processed
properly, then benefits may be denied and your treatment
may suffer. Be sure you have all the forms you need as you
file your claim, and take time to fill in the blanks and to
answer all questions. Medical claims can be held up or
receive nonpayment when people don't follow the instructions. If you need a physician's letter to accompany the form,
be sure you follow through with this, and call your insurance
company after a period of several weeks if there are doubts
as to whether the injury is covered. Most insurance companies have a patient advocate you can call for detailed assistance on a claim.

Q. After trying to juggle a full-time career with the daily pain
and fatigue of fibromyalgia, I've decided to stop work and
apply for disability. Is it difficult to get approved?

A. Because fibromyalgia is extremely difficult to diagnose and
there are no laboratory tests to prove the ailment to a third
party, it's vital that you do your homework before you apply
for disability.

According to federal regulations, to qualify for disability
you must prove that you have a severe impairment that
limits your physical or mental ability to do work activities.
The Social Security disability regulations define disability as
"the inability to do any substantial gainful activity due to
your medical or mental problem." The combined effect of
having multiple impairments is taken into account, which
can be important in many fibromyalgia patients. You must
be unable to do your previous work or any other substantial
gainful activity. Your age and education are considered as
well as your remaining abilities and your work experience.

To start the application for Social Security disability insurance benefits, call your Social Security office. Much of the information may even be provided over the phone or by mail. You will be asked specific questions about how you have trouble with daily activities and you will need to be as specific as you can describing your limitations and why you can't work. You will give the names and addresses of your doctors and the Social Security office will contact each one for records.

Describing your pain by itself will not qualify you for Social Security disability. You must show signs and specific findings of a known medical condition that could be expected to cause your pain. The Social Security staff will consider all your symptoms, including pain, and the medical signs and laboratory tests that give evidence of these. All of this information considered together must allow a conclusion that you are disabled in order for you to be granted disability with benefits. If information that is more detailed is necessary, you may have to be examined by a Social Security approved physician.

It is most common that fibromyalgia patients are not approved, especially with the first application. If you are not approved, you have the right to appeal before a judge who specializes in these cases. Some patients find it necessary to have the help of an attorney during the appeal process. Even though it may increase your costs, the chances of approval of your case are usually better if you have the help of an attorney.

Perhaps one of the most important keys to being approved for disability is having detailed documentation (reports) from your doctors, including psychologists, at the onset of your illness. Have your doctors submit all prescribed medications, therapies, and lifestyle measures that you use to resolve the FMS. You should also be evaluated by a rheumatologist, a doctor who specializes in fibromyalgia and pain-related ailments. This doctor can give a detailed assessment of your impairment, along with the many tests and treatments used in your condition.

Pain is very subjective and difficult to measure, so you'll need to make sure you have statements from all doctors, including psychologists, that further detail your limitations and inability to work. For more details on each step, visit the Social Security Web site (www.ssa.gov/) or call your Social Security office.

Q. I am an editor for a publishing house, so I spend a great deal of time at my computer station. Over the past year, when I get up out of my chair, my back is so sore and stiff. What am I doing wrong?

A. While the aches and muscle pain may be caused by your fibromyalgia, it's possible that at least part of your back pain is caused by excessive stress on the back while you are sitting at work. Sitting in a chair and leaning forward causes higher pressures on the lower spine than sitting straight or standing. Because of this, sitting at a computer terminal for long periods can result in back pain and stiffness.

Using moist heat (a warm shower works very well) and back exercises can give relief of the soreness and stiffness. The exercises will make the back muscles more flexible and stronger, which will help prevent future pain and stiffness. At work, it would help if you could stand up and stretch or walk for a few minutes about every hour. If this is not possible, try stretching while sitting.

Try to use a chair that is comfortable, with arms that can fit under the counter, a firm back support and proper height so that the feet are comfortably flat on the floor. Adjusting the height of the work station to a comfortable level to avoid leaning forward can help avoid fatigue.

RESOURCES

Aids for Arthritis
3 Little Knoll Court
Medford, NY 08055
(609) 654-6918
Web site:
   http://www.aidsforarthritis.com

Alternative Medicine Political
   Action Committee, Inc.
1718 M Street, #205
Washington, DC 20036

American Academy of
   Environmental Physicians
Box CN 1001-2001
New Hope, PA 18938
(913) 642-6062

American Academy of Medical
   Acupuncture
5820 Wilshire Blvd., Suite 500
Los Angeles, CA 90036
213-937-5514
(800) 521-AAMA
Web site:
   www.medicalacupuncture.org

American Academy of Pain
   Management
13947 Mono Way, #A
Sonora, CA 95370
(209) 533-9744
Web site:
   http://www.aapainmanage.org

American Alliance of
   Aromatherapy
P.O. Box 309
Depoe Bay, OR 97341
(800) 809-9850

American Association of
   Alternative Medicine, Inc.
1000 Rutherford Road
Landrum, SC 29356

American Association of
   Naturopathic Physicians
601 Valley Street, Suite 105
Seattle, WA 98109
(206) 298-0126
Web site:
   http://www.naturopathic.org

American Association of Oriental
Medicine
433 Front Street
Catasauqua, PA 18032
(610) 266-1433
Web site:
http://www.aaom.org

American Chiropractic
Association (ACA)
1701 Claredon Blvd.
Arlington, VA 22209
(703) 276-8800
(800) 986-4636
Web site:
www.amerchiro.org

American Chronic Pain
Association
P.O. Box 850
Rocklin, CA 95677
(916) 632-0922

American College of
Rheumatology
60 Executive Park S., Suite 150
Atlanta, GA 30329
(404) 633-3777

American Dietetic Association
(800) 366-1655

American Holistic Medical
Association
6728 Old McLean Village Drive
McLean, VA 22101
(703) 556-9728

American Massage Therapy
Association
820 Davis Street, Suite 100
Evanston, IL 60201
(847) 864-0123
Web site: www.amtamassage.org

American Osteopathic Association
142 East Ontario Street
Chicago, IL 60611
(800) 621-1773

American Physical Therapy
Association
1101 17th Street NW, Suite 1000
Washington, DC 20036
(202) 457-1115

American Preventive Medical
Association
459 Walker Road
Great Falls, VA 22066
(703) 759-0662

American Psychiatric Association
(202) 682-6000

American Psychological
Association
(202) 336-5700

American Self-Help
Clearinghouse
St. Clares–Riverside Medical
Center
25 Pocono Road
Denville, NJ 07834
(201) 625-7101

American Sleep Disorders
  Association
1610 14th Street, Northwest
Suite 300
Rochester, MN 55901
(507) 287-6006

Anxiety Disorders Association of
  America
6000 Executive Blvd., Suite 513
Rockville, MD 20852
(301) 231-9350

Arthritis Foundation
1314 Spring Street
Atlanta, GA 30309
(800) 283-7800
(404) 872-7100

Arthritis Society
250 Floor Street East, Suite 901
Toronto, Ontario
Canada M4W 3P2
(416) 967-1414

Association of Applied
  Psychophysiology and
  Biofeedback
10200 West 44th Avenue,
  Suite 304
Wheat Ridge, CO 80033-2840
(303) 422-8436

Back Pain Association of America
P.O. Box 135
Pasadena, MD 21122
(410) 255-3633
Fax: (410) 255-7338

Biofeedback Certification
  Institute of America
10200 W. 44th Avenue, Suite 304
Wheat Ridge, CO 80033
(303) 420-2902
Web site: www.bcia.org

Fibromyalgia Association
P.O. Box 21988
Columbus, OH 43221-0988
(614) 457-4222
Fax: (614) 457-2729

Fibromyalgia Network
5700 Stockdale Highway, Suite 100
Bakersfield, CA 93309
(805) 631-1950

Help for Incontinent People
P.O. Box 8310
Spartanburg, SC 29305-8310
(864) 579-7900
(800) 252-3337 (BLADDER)

International Chiropractors
  Association (CA)
1110 N. Glebe Road, Suite 1000
Arlington, VA 22201
(703) 528-5000
(800) 423-4690
Web site: www.chiropractic.org

Jaw Joints and Allied
  Musculoskeletal Disorders
  Foundation Inc.
Forsyth's Research Institute
140 Fenway
Boston, MA 02115-3799
(617) 266-2550

Managing Medications
Dept. S
P.O. Box 15329
Stamford, CT 06901
*Send a self-addressed stamped
envelope for information on
recognizing adverse drug
reactions.*

National Arthritis &
Musculoskeletal & Skin
Diseases Information
Clearinghouse
One AMS Circle
Bethesda, MD 20892-3675
(301) 495-4484

National Association
for Holistic
Aromatherapy
P.O. Box 17622
Boulder, CO 80308
Administrative Office
836 Hanley Industrial Court
St. Louis, MO 63144
(888) ASK-NAHA
(324) 963-2071
Fax: (314) 963-4454

National Chronic Fatigue
Syndrome and Fibromyalgia
Association
3521 Broadway, Suite 222
Kansas City, MO 64111
(816) 931-4777

National Commission for the
Certification of Acupuncturists
11 Canal Center Plaza, Suite 300
Alexandria, VA 22314
(703) 548-9004

National Foundation for
Depressive Illness
(800) 239-1263

National Headache Foundation
(800) 843-2256

National Institute of Allergy and
Infectious Diseases
Office of Communications
Bethesda, Maryland
(301) 496-5717

National Institute of Arthritis and
Musculoskeletal and Skin
Diseases
Office of Scientific and Health
Communications
Bethesda, Maryland
(301) 496-8188

National Institute of Dental
Research
Information Office
Bethesda, Maryland
(301) 496-4261

National Institute of Mental
Health Public Inquiries
5600 Fishers Lane, Room 7C-02,
MSC 8030
Bethesda, MD 20892-8030
(301) 496-4000

National Institute of Neurological
   Disorders and Stroke
Office of Scientific and Health
   Reports
Bethesda, Maryland
(301) 496-5751

National Medical Association
   (NMA)
1012 10th Street NW
Washington, DC 20001
(202) 347-1895

National Mental Health
   Association
1021 Prince Street
Alexandria, VA 22314-2971
(703) 664-7722
(800) 969-6642

National Osteopathic Foundation
5775G Peachtree-Dunwoody
   Road, Suite 500
Atlanta, GA 30342
(770) 452-7100

National Qigong (Chi Kung)
   Association
(218) 365-6330
Web site: http://www.nqa.org

National Rehabilitation
   Information Center
8455 Colesville Road, #935
Silver Spring, MD 20910-3319
(800) 346-2742
(301) 588-9284
Fax: (301) 587-1967

North American Spine Society
6300 N. River Road, #115
Rosemont, IL 60018-4231
(708) 698-1630
Fax: (708) 823-8668

Office of Alternative Medicine
   Clearinghouse
P.O. Box 8218
Silver Spring, MD 20907-8218
(888) 644-6226
TTY/TDY: (888) 644-6226
Fax: (301) 495-4957
Web site: altmed.od.nih.gov

Office of Research on Women's
   Health
National Institutes of Health
Bethesda, Maryland
(301) 402-1770

TMJ Association, Ltd.
6418 W. Washington Blvd.
Milwaukee, WI 53213
(414) 259-9334

Government Resources

Americans with Disabilities
(ADA)
Disability Rights Section Mailing
Address:
U.S. Department of Justice
950 Pennsylvania Avenue NW
Civil Rights Division
Disability Rights Section—
NYAVE
Washington, DC 20530
(voice) (800) 514-0301
(TTY) (800) 514-0383
Web site: http://www.usdoj.gov/
crt/ada/adahom1.htm

Centers for Disease Control and
Prevention
(404) 639-5334
Web site: http://www.cdc.gov
Library System, University of
Pittsburgh:
http://www.pitt.edu/~cbw/gov.
html

National Center for
Complementary and
Alternative Medicine
(NCCAM)
National Institutes of Health
Bethesda, MD 20892
Web site:
http://www.nccam.nih.gov
E-mail: info@nccam.nih.gov

Social Security Online
The Official Web site of the Social
Security Administration:
http://www.ssa.gov/

Alternative Medicine Resources

Acupressure and Shiatsu: http://www.acupressure.com/
Alternative Health Benefits Service: http://www.alternativeinsurance.com/
American Academy of Medical Acupuncture:
http://www.medicalacupuncture.org/
American Chiropractic Association: http://www.amerchiro.org
The American Massage Therapy Institute: http://www.amtamassage.org/
Aston-Patterning: http://www.aston-patterning.com/
The Ayurvedic Institute: http://www.ayurveda.com/
The Chiropractic Resource Organization: http://www.chiro.org

The Complete Guide to the Alexander Technique:
    http://www.alexandertechnique.com/
The Feldenkrais Method: http://www.feldenkrais.com/
Global Reiki Network: http://www.reiki.org/
Hellerwork Forum: http://www.alt-med-ed.com/practices/hellerwork.htm
Immunesupport.com: http://www.immunesupport.com/fms_research/
    articles/fm_contag.htm
International Chiropractic Association: http://www.chiropractic.org
Myofascial Release: http://www.myofascial-release.com/
Reflexology: http://www.reflexology.org/
The Rolf Institute: http://www.rolf.org/
Rosen Method Bodywork and Movement: http://www.rosenmethod.org/
The Trager Approach: http://www.trager.com/

REFERENCES AND SUPPORTING RESEARCH

"Alternative Medicine: The Facts." *Consumer Reports* (January 1994): 51.

Antonelli, Mary Ann, M.D., and Robert L. Vawter, M.D. "Nonarticular Pain Syndromes." *Nonarticular Disorders* 91 (February 1992): 95–104.

Arnold, M., et al. A randomized, placebo-controlled, double-blind, flexible-dose study of fluoxetine in the treatment of women with fibromyalgia. *American Journal of Medicine* 112(3) (February 15, 2002): 191–197.

Arthritis Foundation, *Fibromyalgia (Fibrositis)*, 1992.

Barbour, C. "Use of Complementary and Alternative Treatments by Individuals with Fibromyalgia Syndrome." *Journal of the American Academy of Nurse Practitioners* 12(8) (August 12, 2000): 311–316.

Barkhuizen, A. "Pharmacologic Treatment of Fibromyalgia." *Current Pain and Headache Reports* 5(4) (August 2001): 351–358.

Benson, Herbert, M.D., et al. "The Placebo Effect: A Neglected Asset in the Care of Patients." *Journal of the American Medical Association* 232 (1975): 1225–1227.

Benson, H., J. B. Kotch, and K. D. Crasswetter. "Relaxation Response: Bridge Between Psychiatry and Medicine." *Medical Clinics of North America* 61 (1977): 929–938.

Benson, Herbert, M.D., and Eileen M. Stuart, R.N., M.S. *The Wellness Book: The Comprehensive Guide to Maintaining Health and Treating Stress-Related Illness.* New York: Birch Lane Press, 1992.

"Bluer Than Blue." *Involved* (Fall 1993): 2.

Buskila, Dan. "Fibromyalgia, Chronic Fatigue Syndrome, and Myofascial Pain Syndrome." *Current Opinions in Rheumatology* 12(2) (2000): 113–123.

Caldwell, M. S., et al. "Sleep Disturbance, Pain and Emotional Distress in Orofacial Pain Patients." *Journal of Craniomandibular Practice* 19 (April 2001): 106–113.

Cho, Z. H., et al. "New Findings of the Correlation between Acupoints and Corresponding Brain Cortices Using Functional MRI." *Proceedings of the National Academy of Sciences of the United States of America* 95(5) (March 3, 1998): 2670–2673.

Clauw, D. J. "Fibromyalgia: More than Just a Musculoskeletal Disease." *American Family Physician* 52(3) (1995): 843–854.

Crofford, Leslie J., and Daniel J. Clauw. "Fibromyalgia: Where Are We a Decade after the American College of Rheumatology Classification Criteria Were Developed?" *Arthritis and Rheumatism* 46(5) (2002): 1136–1138.

Croft, Peter, Joanna Schollum, and Alan Silman. "Population Study of Tender Point Counts and Pain as Evidence of Fibromyalgia." *British Medical Journal* 309 (September 1994): 696(4).

Dossey, L. *Meaning and Medicinie.* New York: Bantam, 1991.

Dranov, Paula. "Am I Sick or Am I Tired?" *Ladies Home Journal* 106 (September 1989): 120(4).

Duna, George F., M.D., and William S. Wilke, M.D. "Diagnosis, Etiology and Therapy of Fibromyalgia." *Comprehensive Therapy* 19(2) (1993): 60–63.

Dunn, K. S., and A. L. Horgas. "The Prevalence of Prayer as a Spiritual Self-care Modality in Elders." *Journal of Holistic Nursing* 18(4) (December 2000): 337–351.

"Emotions: How They Affect Your Body." *Discover* (November 1984): 35.

"Exercise: A Little Helps a Lot." *Consumer Reports on Health* (August 1994): 89.

Fauci, A. S., E. Braunwald, K. J. Isselbacher, et al., eds. *Harrison's Principles of Internal Medicine.* 14th ed. New York: McGraw-Hill, 1997: 1844, 1900, 1955–1956.

Ferguson, Pamela. *The Self-Shiatsu Handbook.* New York: Perigee Books, 1995.

Ferraccioli, George, et al. "EMG-Biofeedback Training in Fibromyalgia Syndrome." *Journal of Rheumatology* 14 (1987): 820–825.

"Fibromyalgia Unrelenting." *The Back Letter* 9 (May 1994): 60–61.

Garfinkel, M., et al. "Yoga." *Rheumatic Disease Clinics of North America* 26(1) (February 2000): 125–132, x. Review.

Geel, Stanley E. "The Fibromyalgia Syndrome: Musculoskeletal Pathophysiology." *Seminars in Arthritis and Rheumatism* 23 (April 1994): 347–353.

Goleman, D. J. *The Varieties of the Meditative Experience.* New York: Irvington Publishers, 1977.

———. *Mind Body Medicine.* New York: Consumer Reports, 1993.

Griffin, Katherine. "A Whiff of Things to Come." *Health* 6 (November–December 1992): 34.

Hagen, Kathryn. "Feeling Better with Music." *Arthritis Today* 7 (March–April 1993): 19.

Hagglund, K. J., W. E. Deuser, S. P. Buckelew, J. Hewett, and D. R. Kay. "Weather, Beliefs About Weather, and Disease Severity Among Patients with Fibromyalgia." *Arthritis Care and Research* (September 1994): 130–135.

Hansen, C. J., et al. "Exercise Duration and Mood State: How Much Is Enough to Feel Better?" *Health Psychology* 20(4) (July 2001): 267–275.

Hardy, M., et al. "Replacement of Drug Therapy for Insomnia by Ambient Odor." (letter) *Lancet* 346 (1995): 701.

Hollander, L. E. "Sleep Quality, Estradiol Levels, and Behavioral Factors in Late Reproductive Age Women." *Obstetrics and Gynecology* 98 (2001): 391–397.

Ironson, G., et al. "Massage Therapy Is Associated with Enhancement of the Immune System's Cytotoxic Capacity." *International Journal of Neuroscience* 84(1–4) (1996): 205–217.

Keville, Kathi, and Mindy Green. *Aromatherapy: A Complete Guide to the Healing Art.* Berkeley, California: Crossing Press, 1995.

Kjeldsen-Kragh, J., M. Haugen, C. F. Borchgrevink, and O. Forre. "Vegetarian Diet for Patients with Rheumatoid Arthritis." *Clinical Rheumatology* (December 1994): 649.

Kline, Nathan S. *From Sad to Glad.* New York: Ballantine Books, 1974.

Leavitt, F., et al. "Cognitive and Dissociative Manifestations in Fibromyalgia." *Journal of Clinical Rheumatology* 8(2) (2002): 77–84.

Leventhal, L. J., E. G. Boyce, and R. B. Zuerier. "Treatment of Rheumatoid Arthritis with Blackcurrant Seed Oil." *British Journal of Rheumatology* 33 (September 1994): 847–852.

Lipton J. A., and R. A. Dionne, eds. "National Institutes of Health Technology Assessment Conference: Management of Temporomandibular Disorders." *Oral Surgery, Oral Medicine, Oral Pathology, Oral Radiology, Oral Endodontic* 83(1) (1997, Supplement): 49–183.

Locke, Andrew, M.D., and Nicola Gedees, M.D. *The Woman's Guide to Homeopathy.* New York: St. Martin's Press, 1994.

Lorenzen, I. "Fibromyalgia: A Clinical Challenge." *Journal of Internal Medicine* (1994): 199–203.

McClaflin, Richard R., M.D. "Myofascial Pain Syndrome." *Myofascial Pain Syndrome* 96 (August 1994): 56–73.

McIlwain, Harris, M.D., Debra Fulghum Bruce, Joel Silverfield, M.D., Michael Burnette, M.D., and Bernard Germaine, M.D. *Winning with Back Pain.* New York: John Wiley, 1994.

———. *Winning with Chronic Pain.* New York: Prometheus Books, 1994.

Manning F. J., J. A. Barondess, eds. *Changing Health Care Systems and Rheumatic Disease.* Washington, D.C.: National Academy Press, 1996.

Nathan, Ronald G., Thomas E. Staats, and Paul J. Rosch. *The Doctor's Guide to Instant Stress Relief.* New York: G. P. Putnam, 1987.

Novakoski, Frank, A.T.C. "The Benefits of Weight Training." *Living Well Today* (January 1994): 6.

Nye, David A. "Fibromyalgia: A Guide for Patients." http://www.muhealth.org/~fibro/fm-md.html, 1995.

"Optimistic Prognosis for Fibromyalgia Sufferers: Work Disability Uncommon in Decade-Long Study." *The Back Letter* 9 (December 1994): 133(3).

Pei, J., L. Sun, et al. "The Effect of Electro-Acupuncture on Motor Function Recovery in Patients with Acute Cerebral Infarction: A Randomly Controlled Trial." *Journal of Traditional Chinese Medicine* 21(4) (December 2001): 270–272.

Pillemer, Stanley R., M.D. *The Fibromyalgia Syndrome.* New York: Haworth Press, 1994.

"Probing the Mystery of Fibromyalgia." *Health News* 12 (October 1994): 1.

Ray, U. S., et al. "Effect of Yogic Exercises on Physical and Mental Health of Young Fellowship Course Trainees." *Indian Journal of Physiology and Pharmacology* 45(1) (January 2001): 37–53.

Robinson, M. E., J. L. Riley, F. F. Brown, and H. Gremillion. "Sex Differences in Response to Cutaneous Anesthesia: A Double Blind Randomized Study." *Pain* 77 (1998): 143–149.

Roizenblatt, S., et al. "Alpha sleep characteristics in fibromyalgia." *Arthritis and Rheumatism* 44 (2001): 222–230.

Rooks, D. S., et al. "The Effects of Progressive Strength Training and Aerobic Exercise on Muscle Strength and Cardiovascular Fitness in Women with Fibromyalgia: A Pilot Study." *Arthritis and Rheumatism* 47(1) (February 2002): 22–28.

Selye, H. *Stress without Distress.* New York: New American Library, 1975.

Sherman, J. J., et al. "Nonpharmacologic Approaches to the Management of Myofascial Temporomandibular Disorders." *Current Pain and Headache Report* 5(5) (October 2001): 421–431.

Smith, J. D., et al. "Relief of Fibromyalgia Symptoms Following Discontinuation of Dietary Excitotoxins." *Annals of Pharmacotherapy* 35(6) (June 2001): 702–706.

Sorvino, A. R., E. Kalstrom, and Gene G. Abel. "Biofeedback for Musculoskeletal Pain." *Journal of the American Medical Association* 270(22) (December 8, 1993): 2736(1).

Sprott, H., et al. "Microcirculatory Changes over the Tender Points in Fibromyalgia Patients after Acupuncture Therapy (Measured with Laser-Doppler Flowmetry)." *Wiener Klinische Wochenschrift* 112(13) (July 7, 2000): 580–586.

Tuchin, P. J., et al. "A Randomized Controlled Trial of Chiropractic Spinal Manipulative Therapy for Migraine." *Journal of Manipulative and Physiological Therapeutics* 23(2) (February 2000): 91–95.

Vgontzas, A. N., et al. "Middle-Aged Men Show Higher Sensitivity of Sleep to the Arousing Effects of Corticotropin-Releasing Hormone than Young Men: Clinical Implications." *Journal of Clinical Endocrinology and Metabolism* 86(4) (April 2001): 1489–1495.

Wartik, Nancy. "Making Sense of Aromatherapy." *American Health* (October 1995): 73–74.

White, Kevin P., Manfred Harth, and Robert W. Teasell. "Work Disability Evaluation and the Fibromyalgia Syndrome." *Seminars in Arthritis and Rheumatism* 24 (June 1995): 371(10).

Wilke, William S. "Treatment of Resistant Fibromyalgia." *Rheumatic Disease Clinics of North America* (February 1995): 247–260.

Wolfe, Frederick, M.D. "When to Diagnose Fibromyalgia." *Rheumatic Disease Clinics of North America* 20(2) (May 1994): 485–499.

Wurtman, Judith J. "Depression and Weight Gain: The Serotonin Connection." *Journal of Affective Disorders* 29 (1993): 183–192.

Yoshida T., et al. "Non-Invasive Measurement of Brain Activity Using Functional MRI: Toward the Study of Brain Response to Acupuncture Stimulation. *American Journal of Chinese Medicine* 23(3–4) (1995): 319–325.

Yunus, Muhammad B., M.D. "Fibromyalgia Syndrome: A Need for Uniform Classification." *Journal of Rheumatology* 10 (1983): 841–844.

Yunus, M. B., et al. "Relationship between Body Mass Index and Fibromyalgia Features. *Scandinavian Journal of Rheumatology* 31(1) (2002): 27–31.

INDEX

About the Authors

HARRIS H. MCILWAIN, M.D., is board-certified in rheumatology and geriatric medicine, specializing in pain-related diseases. He practices medicine in Florida with the Tampa Medical Group and has written thirteen books on health.

DEBRA FULGHUM BRUCE, M.S., is a medical writer specializing in health and relationships and the author or coauthor of sixty books. She lives in Atlanta, Georgia.